I0434599

GET OFF YOUR BUTT AND DO SOMETHING!

GET OFF YOUR BUTT AND DO SOMETHING!

BEFORE YOU PICKUP A WEIGHT PICK UP THIS BOOK

TOM JACKOBS

Copyright 2010 Tom Jackobs
ISBN 978-0-557-56191-9

This book is for educational and informational purposes for individuals only. Every effort has been made to ensure that the content of this book is accurate. However the publisher and author are not responsible for, nor intend to give, professional advice or service to the individual reader. The ideas in this book are not to be used as a substitute for medical advice from your doctor. Before beginning a fitness routine, you should consult your doctor. The publisher and author are not liable for any loss, damage, or injury allegedly sustained from any suggestions or information contained in this book.

FOREWORD

I spent the first 21 years of my life being the skinny kid with absolutely no athletic abilities. I weighed 125 pounds when I graduated college. Then I got a job and sat on my butt most of the time, ate crap and drank way too much. Believe it or not, I didn't get fat at that point. Then the images of buff guys with ripped abs and bulging biceps started to proliferate in the media and I decided I wanted to look like them. I truly did not make this decision for my own health and wellness but because I didn't want to be the scrawny kid anymore. My two older brothers worked out and were buff, so why couldn't I? I joined a gym, signed a lifetime membership, and received an introduction to the weight machine circuit by the guy who sold me the lifetime membership. It was downhill from there.

I have authored this book for two reasons:

1. I felt like an idiot my first time in the gym and I don't want anyone else to go through that same experience. It shouldn't be that way.
2. I want more people to get off their butts and do something. For themselves.

It is a real shame that I wasted so much time chasing the elusive fitness goal because I didn't know how to actually achieve it. Not to say my desire for a six pack and bulging biceps wasn't achievable, it was. I did eventually achieve the look I so desired but in the beginning, I had no earthly idea what I was doing. I wasted so much time, money and energy on trial and error, listening to advice from strangers and reading too many supplement ads that promised the world in a pill. At that time I didn't know I would eventually own a gym, become a fitness professional and create a company that has helped thousands of people reach their health and fitness goals. But I'm glad I had that experience because it has shaped how I run and operate my fitness business. I don't want anyone who comes into my facility to feel as embarrassed and alone as I felt my first time. We do an awesome job of making our clients and members comfortable and helping them with their commitment. I hope you glean valuable information from this book and if you want to finally **Get Off Your Butt and Do Something**, then I invite you to take advantage of my very special offer at the end of this book. it will be the best investment you'll ever make. If you don't live close to my facility, then I can help you remotely with custom workout programs, meal plans and more.

HOW TO USE THIS BOOK

I've put together a step by step process for you and explained how it works. It is up to you to implement the process and gain the rewards. Quite simply, if you follow these guidelines, you will be successful. At the end of most chapters there are questions and a space for you to write your answers. I STRONGLY suggest you utilize this tool. Once you write down the information, you will solidify the plan in your mind. This will help you to achieve your goals. I know that you can do it!!!

You may also visit the books website www.GetOffYourButtNDoSomething.com for more helpful information and resources to help you along your journey.

TABLE OF CONTENTS

PART ONE

Hopefully, you've picked up this book because you are ready to begin an exciting adventure: *Getting Off Your Butt and Doing SOMETHING... and getting healthier along the way.* You have reason to be excited. What could be more thrilling than giving yourself the gift of a healthier body and adding quality years onto your life? However, starting this vital journey may be overwhelming and you are probably a little intimidated by what's ahead of you. You probably have a lot of questions right now. What is the best way to begin? How much weight can I really expect to lose? How long is it going to take? Which activities should I try? Is it too late for me to ever get in shape? How am I ever going to fit exercise into my already busy schedule?

Pile up too many questions and you can start to feel like throwing in the towel before you even begin! Fortunately, nearly everyone is capable of improving their health and appearance through proper nutrition and exercise, and I do mean EVERYONE. You just need to know how to get started the right way. One of the biggest problems is lacking the knowledge to put a complete program together. That's what I'm going to teach you in this book.

By the time you finish this book, you will have set goals, chosen enjoyable activities, and created a routine. You'll also learn basic ways to improve your eating habits, not by *dieting*, but by understanding how good nutrition is attainable.

In short, you will have a ROADMAP! Once you begin to act on your personal plan, you'll discover how good it feels to improve not only your appearance, but the way you feel physically and emotionally. Then you're on the road to continued health for a life time, never to look in the rearview mirror.

GET ROLLING

Even if you think if feels good to sit on your butt on the couch with a bowl of ice cream, it isn't natural. We are not designed to be sedentary creatures. Until the recent past, physical activity was necessary for human survival. Our bodies are built for, and therefore depend on, continuous movement to stay healthy. It has only been in the last century that large numbers of people in developed nations have become inactive. Modern luxuries such as cars, computers, and televisions, encourage us to sit for long hours each day. This lifestyle change is taking a deadly toll on our country and our world.

According to the Centers for Disease Control and Prevention, inactivity, coupled with a poor diet, will soon be the number one cause of death in the United States. That's not surprising when you consider that two-thirds of American adults are overweight or obese. OVER 66% of 300 Million Americans are overweight or obese, more than 200 million people. Millions are suffering from diseases that can be prevented simply with regular exercise and proper nutrition. I am still shocked and angered by that statistic and quite frankly, you should be too. These numbers also include hundreds of thousands of children – our future! It is now believed that today's population may not live as long as the previous generation due to inactivity and resulting health problems. I was once part of that number. Are you? What are you going to do about it?

> **66% OF AMERICANS ARE OVERWEIGHT**

Despite all of the amazing medical breakthroughs developed by modern scientists, there is no such thing as exercise in a pill. THERE IS NO MAGIC PILL! Nothing can replace physical activity. NOTHING! Need proof? Think about how you feel after sitting on an airplane, sleeping for too long, or being behind a desk all day. Do you feel invigorated or tight and achy?

> **THERE IS NO MAGIC PILL PERIOD!**

When you don't move, your circulation slows down. Some muscles get too tight, while others get loose and flabby. Lack of movement creates all kinds of aches and pains. Now think about how you feel after taking a brisk walk on a nice morning or swimming a few laps. Your blood is pumping a little faster and you feel more limber and energized. There's your proof. When you first start an exercise routine, you may feel sore and stiff, but that will go away with time and training. Flabby arms, a bad heart, and the spare tire around your waist don't go away the more you sit on your butt. Think about what is happening with our bodies with inactivity and poor nutrition, get mad and get motivated.

When I was diagnosed with high blood pressure and high cholesterol at age 30, I got mad and I got motivated. It didn't seem fair that I was having such serious medical issues at such a young age, but the reality is I did it to myself with the choices I made. Now it's time to make different choices, better choices.

BUTT KICKIN': What's your reason for making a change? Write it down right now. That's your motivation and will be key for you to make a positive change in your life and get you back on the road when you veer off in the wrong direction or get lost.

MY MOTIVATION: _____

BENEFITS OF EXERCISE

You already know that a lack of exercise is bad for you. But do you really know just how much regular activity can improve your current physical and mental health? Working out can add quality years to your life by slowing down the aging process in countless ways. One famous study by Harvard University compared nearly 17,000 men and found that as their levels of activity increased their death rates dramatically decreased. Just in case you need additional motivation to put on your sneakers, here's a partial list of what you can expect to happen when you stick to a solid exercise program:

- Weight loss, trimmer appearance
- Improved skin tone
- Increased sex drive
- Reduced stress
- Improved mood and self-esteem
- Better, more restful, sleep
- Increased energy
- Better circulation
- Stronger immune system
- Lower Blood Pressure
- Less risk of osteoporosis
- Less chance of developing deadly cancers, including colon and breast cancers
- Reduced risk of stroke
- Reduced risk of heart disease

There is growing evidence that regular exercise can ward off mental decline in older adults as well.

BUTT KICKIN': But do you really need this list? Look at what's going on right now in your life: Do you think it would be improved if you moved better, didn't get tired so easily, or weren't so edgy? List three benefits you want.

1.

2.

3.

FIGURING OUT YOUR DESTINATION

You may think be thinking, "I already know where I want to be. I want to lose weight by working out and eating better." That's a wish, not a goal. Setting a goal is something that takes thought and planning. Think about our roadmap analogy, "I want to go on a road trip" doesn't get you to where you want to be, it may get you moving, but are you going in the right direction? In this chapter, we are going to discuss how you can devise goals that are both specific and realistic.

First, let's talk about setting specific goals. These goals must be targets that you can objectively measure. Don't just say "I want a flatter stomach and smaller thighs." You need to be more specific because you can't measure subjective ideas. After all, your stomach may look larger after a big meal, or suddenly flatter in the right pair of pants. That doesn't mean you have taken a step backwards or made real progress. Sometimes, your mood will affect your perception of how you look.

So instead, you might say, "I want to get my body fat down to 20% in 12 weeks" or "I want to be able to walk two miles on the treadmill in 26 minutes by the end of next month." These are specific targets that you can work towards while measuring your progress. You should always set a specific timeframe for meeting your goals. Otherwise, there is no urgency to meeting your goals. Be careful not to make your goal too far out in the future or you may never start as you may think you have plenty of time to complete it.

This is not to say you shouldn't have long term goals, but you must have shorter term goals which break your longer goals into manageable pieces. As with a road trip, you will need to plan your stops along the way.

As an example, you might want to lose 25 pounds over the next three months, or 50 pounds over the course of six months. These goals are reasonable and are specific. However, if you are new to exercising, you might find it hard to keep focused on the same target for three months, let alone six months or a year. Create short-term goals, or benchmarks, along the way to help you stay motivated. Perhaps you could focus on losing eight pounds during the first month. Once you've reached that goal, reward yourself with an appropriate reward, revaluate your progress and set the next goal. Repeat this cycle until you've reached your long-term goals. By celebrating each small step, it will be easier to chart your progress and you'll maintain your motivation and excitement as you work towards your larger goals.

Now that you have set specific goals, you may be very excited to get started. However, take another look at them and make sure they are realistic. With hard work and determination, you will be able to make major, positive changes in how your body looks, feels, and functions. However, just because you decide you want to lose 50 pounds, it doesn't mean that your body will cooperate. Your goal weight should be realistic for your height and frame. Goals that involve making big changes are thrilling. Just be careful that your goals don't cross the line between "ambitious" and "impossible."

Also, when setting your goals, don't get sucked in by ads or magazine pictures featuring pumped-up men or women wearing size zero jeans. For most of us, looking like airbrushed supermodels will remain impossible, no matter how hard we work. Your goals should focus on becoming healthier and fitter. If you make your body stronger, your outward appearance is bound to improve. Just don't get it backwards and put appearance before health. An unrealistic quest for perfection will only make you more likely to fall prey to extreme diets and routines that will leave you feeling like you have failed, or even worse, cause an injury or illness.

When setting your goals, remember that safe weight loss programs will help you lose more fat than lean muscle. Therefore, you should strive for a weight loss of one to two pounds per week. More than that will be counterproductive. Be patient with yourself. Becoming fitter is wonderful, thrilling, and well worth the effort, but it is going to take time.

BUTT KICKIN': Setting goals is an important part of your journey to better health. Focus on setting both long-term and short-term (or benchmark) goals. Make sure your plans are not too easy or unrealistic. Remember to set goals that are challenging, not unachievable.

MY SPECIFIC GOAL: _____

MY TIME FRAME: _____

REACHING YOUR GOALS

At this point, you should have a good idea about your specific and realistic goals as you embark on your new fitness plan. Now you need to figure out how you are going to achieve those goals by incorporating your plan into your daily life. Here's a list of ways to keep motivated and on track:

- Write your goals on a piece of paper and hang it where you will see it every day. If you start to ignore your posted goals because you see them every day, and you will, post them someplace else, like on your computer or bathroom mirror. Change the location so they don't lose their impact and continually stay top of mind

- Work your short term goals into your daily routine. Figure out what you can do EVERYDAY to reach your objectives. Even on days when you do not workout, make choices that remind you of your fitness plan. Maybe you walk instead of taking an elevator, drink all of your water, or discover a healthy recipe. Whatever you do, make everyday a step toward achieving your goals. At the end of the day, ask yourself "how did I do today?" If the answer is not positive, then figure out how you can make tomorrow a better day.

- Chart your progress. Create a weekly workout plan (which will be explained in an upcoming chapter) and track each workout as you complete it. It is very satisfying to see the number of checkmarks grow! Also, keep track of improvements in your strength, endurance, and weight. If you are trying to lose weight, take your measurements now, then retake them every four weeks to monitor your progress.

- Decide how you will reward yourself for reaching your short-term and long-term goals. These rewards do not have to be large or detrimental to your bank account. Just don't reward yourself with a big, fattening meal or desert, because that will only reinforce negative, emotional eating. Make your rewards complement your goals, such as scheduling a golf lesson or getting a massage.

BUTT KICKIN': Create your own plan of action and the reward you will give yourself for completing your daily plan. Don't make the reward food based!

MY DAILY ACTION PLAN: _____

MY REWARD FOR COMPLETION: _____

EXCUSES, EXCUSES

You know exercise is good for you, even before reading the list of the many ways that exercise benefits your body. Perhaps you feel motivated and ready to workout now. Ask yourself what has stopped you from acting sooner? Really consider why you have not exercised regularly. Make a list. You need to know exactly what has been holding you back, because those nagging "reasons" will pop up again and again on days when exercising seems like too much trouble. You need to be ready to face your excuses.

Maybe you think working out is boring or you don't like the idea of going to a gym. Perhaps you feel too tired after leaving work. The couch seems so much more inviting than the treadmill. If you are like many adults, you think that you just don't have enough time. After all, you rush around in the morning, work all day, maybe take care of the kids at night and before you know it, the day is over. You probably can barely find five minutes to have a cup of coffee and read the newspaper, so how are you going to fit exercise into your already hectic schedule?

Be honest with yourself. Until now, if you had magically received 30 more minutes in each day, would you really have spent it exercising? Probably not. You will never fit exercise into your schedule until you make it a *priority*. Now, think about your fitness goals again. We are talking about your health! You can't afford not to find time for the preservation of your life. Besides, what good are all of those activities that fill your day if you are not healthy enough to enjoy them?

Since you're never going to be given more time, you'll have to deliberately schedule time for exercise. Some people prefer to get up early and exercise in the morning, some stay-at-home parents squeeze in workouts during the baby's naptime, while others like to hit the gym before heading home after work. There are no "best" times to exercise. The "best" time is any time that you'll be able to fit it in. Some experts think people who workout in the morning are more likely to stick to their routines because it is the first thing they do each day. Waiting to exercise can be an invitation for roadblocks, such as those unexpected family and work responsibilities that pop-up, forcing you to change your plans. If you are going to workout later in the day, that is fine. Just make sure you don't get sidetracked. Finding a good time for exercise might take some trial and error. After a few workouts, decide if the times are working for you. If not, try a new schedule.

Put your exercise sessions on your calendar and make it a priority, just like you would your daughter's soccer game, a doctor's appointment, or a sales meeting. Finding an exercise partner can also be a good way to keep your workout appointments, because most people are less likely to blow off a workout if they know someone is waiting for them. Whatever workout time you choose, share your new plan with your family and friends and let them know it is important to you. Ask them to support and respect your goals and not infringe on your important exercise time.

Get that notion out of your head that it takes hours a day to get fit. It doesn't. If you can squeeze 30 minutes of good quality exercise in 6 out of 7 days a week you will be well on your way to achieving your goals. That's 3 hours a week. If you tell me you can't spend 3 hours on improving the quality of your life then I call bull on you. If this is your attitude, please put this book down and take it back to the bookstore and get your money back because you are clearly not ready to get off your butt and do something! Nothing get's those nonexistent hairs on the back of my neck standing up straight more than someone saying they don't have 3 hours a week to improve the quality of their life. If you want it bad enough you'll find those 3 hours. I got up at 5:00 a.m. every morning to ensure I would lose weight and get healthy. I planned my meals meticulously each and every week and I was working a full time job and traveling about 50% of the time. So don't tell me you don't have time, if you want it bad enough you'll make the time.

As far as being too tired to exercise, try a little experiment with yourself. When you feel like you are dragging and want to lie down, force yourself to do 20 minutes of aerobic exercise. You don't have to do anything major, just get your heart rate up and break a sweat. Even a walk around the neighborhood will work. Chances are you will feel totally rejuvenated and energized when you're done. Exercise activates growth hormones and stimulates our nervous system, so it can be a great pick-me-up after a long day.

BUTT KICKIN': It's important to identify the roadblock that will potentially hold you back from reaching your goals right now. In doing so, you will recognize what they are and determine a way around the block. So write down what potential roadblocks might come up and determine, right now, how you're going to stare them down!.

What's Holding me Back

Roadblock | How I'll blast through it

_____ | _____

_____ | _____

MYTHS

Bad information sometimes stops people from starting an exercise program. There are as many exercise myths as there are excuses. Don't fall prey to exercise myths, including these:

- "Exercise takes too much time." We've already covered this excuse. The truth is that exercise should not take more than 30 to 60 minutes a day. Furthermore, any exercise is better than none. Even walking for as little as an hour a week has been shown to reduce the risk of heart disease.

- "Exercising will make you tired." Exercise will not make you more tired during the day. In fact, many people who workout regularly report increased energy.

- "Some people just aren't athletic." Regular exercise is for everyone, no matter if you are an athlete or not. Many exercises, including walking and simple strength exercises, require no special ability.

- "If you start exercising and then stop, your muscles will turn into fat." Wrong again. Working out now will not make you fatter if you stop later. Fat and muscle are two completely different types of tissue. One will not turn into the other. However, if you stop working out, but continue to take in the same number of calories, you will gain fat and your muscles will atrophy.

- "Women who lift weights will get bulky." Strength training is an essential part of a well-rounded fitness plan. While lifting weights will make you stronger and firmer (that's a good thing!), it will not cause women to "bulk up." Women do not have the genetic ability to form huge muscles because they don't have enough testosterone. End of story.

WHAT'S IN YOUR GYM BAG?

OK, you are almost ready to hit the gym. But first, a quick word about what should be in your gym bag. First and foremost, you need good shoes. Not the shoes that you have had since high school that are currently collecting dust in your closet. Not the casual sneakers you have worn to the mall for the last two years. If you're serious about getting fit, you need serious shoes. Serious shoes don't have to cost a fortune, but they do have to fit right and provide stability for the type of exercise you are going to be performing. You should expect to pay market price for a solid pair of athletic shoes.

It's best to shop for shoes later in the day. Your feet will have swollen since the morning. If you require any type of orthotic when you exercise, take it to the store so you can make sure the shoes will fit comfortably. You should also wear athletic socks when trying on gym shoes, because they are thicker than other socks and you need to make sure your shoes are not going to be too tight.

Once you have found a pair of shoes you want to try on, don't make a choice based on looks alone, no matter how sharp those shoes look on your feet! The heel should be snug, but not too tight. You should have about a thumb's width between your longest toe and the end of the toe box. Try on both shoes and lace them all the way up. Now walk, run, and jump around a bit. (Don't mind the curious onlookers. You need to make sure the shoes will be comfortable.) While you're moving, the shoes should bend at the ball of the foot. Most importantly, banish any thoughts of "breaking-in" a pair of sneakers. Don't make the mistake of thinking the shoes will eventually stretch or conform to your foot. Athletic footwear should feel comfortable immediately. I always recommend going to a specialty shoe store as the clerks are much more educated on shoe fit for every purpose than in a department store or a general sporting goods store.

The rest of what you put into your gym bag is up to you. It will vary according to what exercises you plan to perform and how much stuff you like to carry around. Here's a partial list of common items that can make your workout more effective and pleasurable:

- Your gym membership card

- Your workout program and tracking log book

- Pen or Pencil

- Music player with headphones

- Toiletries, shower shoes and extra clothing if you plan on showering

- Plastic grocery bags that can hold your sweaty clothes and keep them from getting the inside of your bag wet (make sure you don't let them sit in the bag overnight or they'll start to look like a science experiment... and smell like one too!)

- Water bottle, cleaned from last use.

- Towels if the gym does not have a towel service. You'll need one for showering and one for wiping down equipment

- Your post workout recovery drink or a healthy snack for after your workout (more on this later) especially if it will be a while until your next meal.

- Heart rate monitor

CHOOSING A GYM

There are many good reasons to join a gym. First, if you go to the gym, you are going to exercise. There is nothing else to do or to distract you. Plus, you'll have access to more professional exercise equipment than you will ever be able to accumulate at home. Finally, you can learn a lot about proper exercise by spending time talking to and observing instructors, trainers, and knowledgeable members. However, all of the reasons in the world won't keep you going to the gym if you are not comfortable with the facility you pick. Here are some things to consider before buying a membership:

- Location, location, location! Pick a gym that is as close as possible to your home or work. If the gym is too far away, you will not go consistently. It will be too easy to make the excuse that you don't have time to make it there and back. You may want to pick a gym that is on your way to work. This will make it easier to schedule your workouts around your work schedule.

- Look at the variety of equipment. As someone who is new to fitness, you will only need the basics. Still, there should be several different types of cardiovascular machines, a decent supply of free weights, and various simple weight machines so you do not get bored, as well as all sorts of fun fitness toys like balls and bands. You don't need a lot of machines to get a good workout. Using too many machine-based exercises may in fact do more harm than good, if not used properly.

- See how crowded the gym gets. Take a tour of facility at the same time you plan to use it. If people are waiting in line to get on the elliptical machine, you should probably go somewhere else. Your workout time is limited and you don't want to spend it standing around. When the American Council on

Exercise polled people about why they stopped going to the gym, nearly half said overcrowding.

- Is the place clean? Try out a few machines and see how easy they are to operate. Are they smooth or rusty? Do the seats look new or are they patched with duct tape? Is there plenty of access to cleaning spray and paper towels so you can wipe down machines? Check out the locker rooms. Gyms can be a breeding ground for all kinds of disgusting things. You don't want to be grossed out when you work out.

- How large is the gym? Some people really love huge sports complexes with all of the bells and whistles. If this is important to you, go for it. However, many beginners prefer a smaller, less overwhelming gym that provides a supportive environment where they can get to know the employees and other members. The gym I operate is around 4,000 square feet and enables my staff and me to get to know each member. We really cater to those who have never worked out before.

- Find out what extra services the gym provides. Do you want a towel service or would you rather bring your own? Some people will require a daycare or kids gym. Others may be interested in a gym that also provides spa services, fitness classes, personal training or nutritional counseling.

Once you join a gym, going inside as a member for the first time may be intimidating. Some people immediately start comparing themselves to the size 0 model on the elliptical or the buff bodybuilder standing near the weight rack flexing in the mirror. Don't do this to yourself. There will always be someone stronger, bigger, smaller, lighter, or heavier than you. You have come to the gym to improve yourself, not to compete. If you are nervous about working out in a public place, try going with a friend or during off-peak hours when there are not as many people around.

When using the equipment, never be embarrassed about not knowing how to operate something. Just ask someone. Everybody was a beginner at one point; no one was born knowing how to use a leg press machine. Finally, don't assume people are staring at you. They are most likely too busy checking them*selves* in the mirror to care what you are doing. After all, do you *really* care what they are doing?

BUTT KICKIN': Now its time to identify which gyms you want to visit for a tour. Of course if you live in Houston I invite you to come visit mine. Do an internet search for gyms either near your home or work. Make a list here and plan your visits.

GYMS NEAR HOME:

1.

2.

3.

GYMS NEAR WORK:

1.

2.

3.

HIRING A FITNESS PROFESSIONAL

Hiring a fitness professional can be one of the best investments you make if you are serious about getting into shape. There are many benefits to having a professional to guide your workouts. There is a big difference between a personal trainer and a fitness professional. A true fitness professional will be more than a drill instructor, barking out orders and counting reps. Fitness professionals serve as your teacher and educate you about how your body works and proper exercise forms. This is crucial if you are just starting out. Fitness professionals also alleviate the feeling of being overwhelmed that many experience the first time they go to a gym. It is common for people to not like going to a gym because they feel intimidated by all of the unfamiliar looking equipment. They are scared that they will use it incorrectly and look foolish or even worse, hurt themselves. A fitness professional can take away the fear of the unknown. I wish I had hired a fitness professional when I first joined a gym. I would have saved years of trial and error.

A fitness professional can also keep you motivated by safely pushing you further than you would push yourself. If you find yourself frequently skipping important exercises that you don't like, you should consider hiring a coach. You can't cheat if someone else is keeping count. Furthermore, most people are also less likely to skip workouts if they have paid for an appointment.

The right fitness professional can be a great source of information and motivation. Even if you can't afford to have a trainer several times a week, there are ways to make the sessions fit into your budget. If the session rate sounds high, ask if they can customize something that fits within your budget. Some fitness professionals also provide discounts if you sign up with a friend or relative. Even if you don't use a trainer on a regular basis, a few sessions at the start of your new exercise routine can be invaluable. After that, you can check in with your trainer ever few weeks to help chart your progress and reevaluate your routine.

Whether you want to establish a long-term relationship with a fitness professional, or just sign up for a few learning sessions, there are questions you should ask before making a financial commitment. Just because someone looks the part of a fitness professional, doesn't mean they have the education to keep you safe and help you reach your goals. So absolutely ask these questions to someone you're considering hiring. Since I received my fitness professional certification, I have NEVER been asked to provide proof of it, even though I keep my certificates handy.

- What is your educational background? Do you have a degree in physical education, exercise science, or a related field? This may not be necessary, but it is a sign that the trainer has been educated in how the body moves.

- Are you certified? There are many types of certifications. Some require college degrees and most require that students pass an exam. The American Council on Exercise (ACE), Aerobics and Fitness Association of American (AFFA), and the American College of Sports Medicine (ACSM) are just some of the reputable national certification programs. Keep in mind that a certification is not a guarantee of education, as there are plenty of certification "mills" that will hand out a certification to anyone who pays $49 over the internet.

- How long have you been a fitness professional? Proper education is crucial, but hands-on experience is the best way to learn how to be a good trainer. Ideally, your trainer will have both education and experience.

- Will you help me to devise programs that I can follow on days that I workout on my own? This is important because unless you want to hire a trainer to be with you five times a week, you'll be working out mostly on your own.

- Can you meet my particular needs? This is whatever special conditions you may have, including past injuries, high blood pressure, etc. In order to keep your workouts safe, your trainer must know what exercises may be dangerous and which ones will help you build strength in your weak areas.

- Do you offer a money-back guarantee? This may sound odd, but it's important. You're about to invest a serious amount of money and you should know that the program you're signing up for is going to help you reach your goals. By having a written guarantee, you will know exactly what you need to do to reach your goals and what the fitness professional is going to do to help you reach them.

- When are you available? The best trainer in the world will not be able to help you get into shape if you have opposite schedules and time commitments. You can also ask any potential trainer how many clients they are currently seeing. If your trainer's schedule is too full, how can you expect him/her to make time for you?

You should be wary of any fitness professional who does not ask you about your goals, medical background, and previous workout history. Your trainer should also know how to take your blood pressure, heart rate, and body composition, and how to give a fitness assessment test. Finally, once you start working with a trainer, see how much they listen to you and whether or not they are concerned about teaching you to work out independently. You won't always be working out with their guidance.

Be careful of any trainer who immediately starts you out on exercise without first at least assessing what you are capable of doing and understanding if you've ever exercised before or if you have any medical issues.

You also have to do your part in this relationship. Remember that your trainer is a paid professional, not your new best friend, so keep you workouts somewhat businesslike. Don't be late, whine about the routine, or discuss the more intimate details of your life. However, you need to have friendly rapport with your trainer, so don't be afraid to switch fitness professionals if you feel uncomfortable for any reason or simply don't feel like you "click." You should be able to enjoy and look forward to your sessions.

BUTT KICKIN': The best way to find a fitness professional is to ask friends for a recommendation, you can also locate one through the certifications holders such as (ACE, AFAA, ACSM, NASM).

List 3 Fitness Professions to Interview:

1.

2.

3.

YOUR HOME GYM

Even if you belong to a gym, there are benefits to owning home exercise equipment. For starters, there are some days that you may be pressed for time. Not having to travel to the gym can mean the difference between skipping a workout and managing to squeeze in 30 minutes for exercise.

Your home gym can consist of just a few pieces of equipment. You'll want items that allow you to get some form of aerobic, anaerobic, and flexibility training. A bare bones home gym might not require more than a few workout videos, some light, medium, and heavy dumbbells, a couple of different strength resistance bands and a yoga mat. If you want to purchase a machine for cardio or strength training, carefully consider what you like to use when you are at the gym. There is no sense in buying a treadmill if you hate cardio equipment. Perhaps you would be better off with a step for step aerobics.

No matter what you decide to purchase, make sure you put it in a place in your home where you enjoy spending time. Chances are your stationary bike will just collect dust if you put it in the dark corner of a basement. Plus, if you can see your equipment, you are more likely to use it for more than just hanging wet clothes..

If you travel a lot, then create an easy exercise travel kit. All you really need is a few different strength exercise bands and your body weight. When I travel I rarely go to the hotel gym, I can do a complete strength and cardio workout in the comfort and privacy of my hotel room. You just need some creativity or guidance.

There are many products on the market in all price ranges. You'll want to steer clear of buying gadgets just because the advertisements make great sounding promises. Here are some red flags to look for when purchasing any fitness products:

- Don't believe any claim that you can drop pounds or inches in a short period time. Catch phrases in these types of ads often include promises like "lose 10 pounds in 10 days" or "see inches melt away."

- Don't believe ads that insist that a piece of exercise equipment will allow you to receive maximum results with little daily effort. You will not ever achieve washboard abs by only working out 7 minutes a day. I know this from experience!

- Disregard any "before" and "after" pictures. These photos are almost always misleading and were not achieved by only using the advertised product.

- Don't buy equipment from a company that you have never heard of without doing your homework. Before purchasing, find out how the company treats its customers. When you call the toll-free number, are customer service representatives helpful? What is the return and warranty policies?

Having a few pieces of home exercise equipment can be a great idea. However, keep in mind that going to a gym allows you to incorporate a wider variety of exercises, which is important to overall fitness. Gyms also are great places for the beginner to learn how to properly perform exercises, and a great place to meet other health conscious people interested in improving their life.

BUTT KICKIN': Create a list of items you want for your home gym or your travel workout kit.

1.

2.

3.

4.

5.

SHOULD YOU SEE YOUR DOCTOR BEFORE GETTING OFF YOUR BUTT?

Before you begin reaping the benefits of an exercise program, you may need to set up an appointment with your doctor, especially if you have been sedentary for more than a year. You should also see a doctor if you answer yes to any of the following questions.

- Has your doctor ever said you have a heart condition and should only do activity recommended by a doctor?

- Do you feel pain in your chest when you do physical activity?

- In the past month, have you had chest pain when you were not doing physical activity?

- Do you lose your balance because of dizziness or do you ever lose consciousness?

- Do you suffer from shortness of breath at mild exertion or have difficulty breathing?

- Do you have a bone or joint problem that could be made worse by a change in your physical activity?

- Is your doctor currently prescribing drugs for your blood pressure or heart condition?

- Do you know of any other reason why you should not do physical activity?

- Are you above 40 years of age and not currently physically active?

- Has your doctor ever said you have high blood pressure (140/90 mm Hg or above)?

- Have you ever taken any medication to lower your blood pressure?

- Has your doctor ever said you have high blood cholesterol (200 Total or above)?

- Do you have diabetes or high blood sugar?

- Do you currently smoke or have you quit in the last 6 months?

BUTT KICKIN': Visit your doctor and get a report of the lab results. Document your health numbers and any restrictions your doctor gave you here.

Blood Pressure:

Cholesterol:

Blood Sugar:

Restrictions:

PART TWO

NOW YOU'RE 'ALMOST' READY TO DO SOMETHING!

THE FIRST TEST

Your goals are set, your future workout sessions are on the calendar, you've got new sneakers on your feet, and you've arrived at the gym. Now what? Many people begin their first workout by automatically jumping on a treadmill or sitting down at a random machine and starting to push and/or lift weight. This haphazard, uneducated approach to exercising can severely slow down your progress and even lead to injury. That is exactly what I did and I spent 5 more years paying dues on a gym membership I didn't use! First, you need to assess where you are in terms of your fitness level.

A personal trainer can guide you through a fitness assessment test (really consider this.) Even if you do not have a personal trainer, many gyms will provide these tests for their members during special events or upon request. Our gym does this for all of our members once a month, but we're pretty special that way! However, if you are working out alone, you can perform most of the tests yourself. Either way, take the time for a full assessment. After all, you'll never know how far you've come if you don't know your exactly where you started.

First, begin by taking your measurements, preferably with help from someone else. If you decide to do it yourself, stand in front of a full length mirror so you can make sure the measuring tape is always pulled straight and not sagging. Measure in the following places and record the numbers:

- Shoulders: across the widest part of your shoulders, above where your arms begin

- Chest: keep your chest at its normal size, don't stick it out or take deep breaths. Men wrap the tape measure around their chest, right under the armpits. Women should measure at the fullest part of the breast.

- Biceps: around the widest part of your upper arm, do one measurement relaxed and another flexed.

- Stomach: right across your belly button above the waist, right around the love handles, if you have them (I know, I know... this is no one's favorite place to measure). And do NOT suck your stomach in or make it protrude out unnaturally.

- Hips: around the fullest part of your buttocks

- Thighs: around the upper leg, extend your hands down the side of your leg and measure where your finger tips are.

- Calves: around the thickest part while flexed by pointing the toe and raising the heel

Plan to take your measurements again in about 4 weeks in the exact same spots.

Now, record your weight. But remember to keep this measurement in perspective. Too often people obsess over the numbers on the scale. While it is important to know how much you weigh in order to chart your progress, it is only one tool in assessing your overall fitness. When making progress, your weight is not as much of an indicator of success than how your pants fit.

The next tests will help you determine your fitness level. Fitness is described in many different ways. However, most experts agree that there are five basic components to fitness, which you will test before you start your regular exercise program. They are:

- Muscular Strength: The greatest amount of force a muscle or muscle group can exert in a single effort.

- Muscular Endurance: The ability to hold a position for a particular period of time, or repeat a movement for an extended period of time.

- Cardio Respiratory Function: This is the ability to do continuous, moderately strenuous activity. During aerobic exercise, your cardio respiratory system (heart and lungs) work together to supply oxygen to your body.

- Flexibility: The ability to move a joint through its full range of motion. This is also referred to as how limber someone is.

- Body Composition: This test tells you what percentage of your body is made up of fat, instead of lean muscle and other tissue. Your weight is not nearly as important as your body fat composition.

OK, it is finally time to get moving. Before beginning the following tests, warm-up for at least five minutes by performing some type of gentle aerobic exercise, like walking on a treadmill or marching in place.

Upper Body Strength and Stamina: Nothing gives you a better idea of your upper body strength and endurance like good old fashioned push-ups. Begin by doing as many push-ups as you can without stopping. Rest for one minute. Repeat. Now write down how many reps (that's short for repetitions) you performed in each set. If you could only do a handful on the first set, you should try to build strength. If you are able to do more than a dozen or so during the first set, but can only manage a few on the second set, it's time to work on stamina.

When doing a push-up, keep your hands in line with your shoulders and your arms straight. Before lowering your body, you should be in a straight line from the top of your head to your heels. Keep your abdominal area tight and pulled in. Your hands and feet will be supporting your weight. Maintaining your form, with eyes straight ahead, slowly bring your chest to about 3" off the floor (about the size of a fist). Before your chest touches the floor, push yourself back up. Women can do these standard push-ups or modified push-ups. In a modified push-up, the form is the same, but before lowering your body the first time, bend and rest both knees on the ground. Cross you legs and slowly lower your body.

These charts give you a general idea of upper body strength, based on the number of push-ups you could do in one set:

MEN

Age	20-29	30-39	40-49	50-59	60 +
Kicking Butt	>47	>41	>34	>31	>30
Pretty Good Butt Kickin'	35-46	30-40	21-33	18-30	17-29
Butt Kickin'	20-34	17-29	11-20	9-17	6-16
Needs a Kick in the Butt	>19	>16	>10	>8	>5

WOMEN

Age	20-29	30-39	40-49	50-59	60 +
Kicking Butt	>30	>30	>25	>21	>19
Pretty Good Butt Kickin'	23-29	22-30	18-24	15-20	13-18
Butt Kickin'	12-22	10-21	8-17	7-14	5-12
Needs a Kick in the Butt	<11	<9	<7	<6	<4

Lower Body Strength and Stamina: This test will be performed by doing squats. Stand with your feet about shoulder-width apart. Keep your back straight and squat down slowly until your thighs are almost parallel to the floor. If you need a physical indicator of how far to go, place a chair behind you and squat just until your buttocks touch, or almost touch, the seat. Look down at your feet and make sure your knees are not extending beyond your toes. You should not feel any pain in your knees, if you do then stop the exercise and check your form. Lift your head, pause, and then rise back up as slowly as you can. You have completed one full squat. Now, do as many as you can at the same slow speed until you have reached exhaustion. Record the number.

MEN

Age	20-29	30-39	40-49	50-59	60 +
Kicking Butt	>40	>35	>29	>25	>22
Pretty Good Butt Kickin'	35-39	30-34	25-28	21-24	19-21
Butt Kickin'	29-34	23-29	18-25	13-20	11-18
Needs a Kick in the Butt	>28	>22	>17	>12	>10

WOMEN

Age	20-29	30-39	40-49	50-59	60 +
Kicking Butt	>33	>27	>22	>18	>17
Pretty Good Butt Kickin'	29-32	23-26	18-21	13-17	14-16
Butt Kickin'	21-28	15-22	10-17	7-12	5-13
Needs a Kick in the Butt	>20	>14	>8	>6	>4

Cardio Endurance: This test will tell you how hard your heart has to work while you are exercising and how quickly it returns to its normal, resting rate. In this test, you will measure your heart rate before, during, and after three minutes of moderate aerobic exercise. If you take this test after the others, wait a few minutes before you begin so that your body has a chance to fully cool down. To measure your heart rate, count your pulse for 15 seconds before you start exercising. Multiply that number by four and write down the result. Now, begin to exercise at a pace that feels a bit strenuous, but does not leave you gasping for breath. You should still be able to talk. Perform this aerobic exercise for three minutes. Take your pulse and record the number. Wait and rest for one minute. Take your pulse and right down the number again.

As you become more fit, all three of these numbers should start to decrease. The lower resting heart rate (taken before you start) will mean that your heart is becoming more efficient and pumping more blood with fewer beats. During exercise, your heart will be better able to handle aerobic stress. After exercise, your heart rate will return to normal at a faster rate, meaning it will be able to recover more quickly from exertion.

Flexibility: Many people forget about flexibility and skip stretching at the end of a workout. However, exercises that build strength tend to shorten muscle, which limits your range of motion. A limited range of motion can contribute to an increased risk of injury, so never forget to stretch. You can test your current flexibility by sitting on the floor with your legs stretched out in front of you and your feet hip width apart. Put one hand on top of the other and place them on the floor between your legs. Keeping your back straight and slowly extend your hands towards your feet. See how far you get. Perhaps you can go all the way past your feet. Maybe you only made it to the lower shin. Write down your results. The next time you test, you will hopefully be able to go past the point you are at now.

Body Composition: There are several ways to test the percentage of your body that is composed of fat instead of lean tissue. The most readily available methods are calculating your body mass index (BMI) and skin-fold measurements. The BMI only provides a very general number and does not make allowances for various body types. For example, many athletes would be considered obese using this method, because they are physically heavy for their height. The BMI calculation does not take into account that their weight is mostly muscle, not fat. For this reason, I don't like to use the BMI scale. Still, for most people the BMI method will give a rough guide to your general composition. To calculate BMI you divide your weight in pounds by your height in inches squared and multiply it by 703. So, here's how a 220 pound man who is 75" tall would calculate his BMI:

$$BMI = (220/(75*75)) * 703 = 20$$

The skin-fold measurement is more accurate in terms of allowing you to separate your lean weight with your actual fat weight. Calipers are the instrument used to measure body fat and can be purchased on-line (visit the resources section of www.GetOffYourButtNDoSomething.com). Body fat calipers measure the thickness of a fold of skin and its underlying layer of fat. Certain locations on the body will give a fairly accurate way to estimate your total percentage of body fat. Calipers can be inexpensive and usually come with instructions. But it is best to have a professional perform these measurements for the most accurate result.

When testing your body fat, the minimum percent of body fat that is considered safe is 5% for men and 12% for women (this is where many athletes keep their body fat). A percentage of body fat that is too high will increase the risk of diseases and chronic illnesses. A dangerously high level for men is more than 25% body fat and 32% for women. The healthy zone for men is from 12% to 17% and women should stay between 17% and 27%.

Repeat these tests every four weeks. With steady work, all of your numbers should begin moving in the right direction, and if they aren't then something needs to change.

BUTT KICKIN': Write down your evaluation numbers here.

Pushups:

Squats:

Flexibility:

Body Composition:

THE KEY TO FITNESS: PERFORMING A VARIETY OF EXERCISES

People who are new to fitness often pick one type of exercise they enjoy and it becomes their entire workout routine. There are a lot of people, especially women, who go to the gym religiously to use

> CRAZY: [KREY-ZEE]
> DOING THE SAME THING
> AGAIN AND AGAIN
> EXPECTING A
> DIFFERENT RESULT!

the treadmill or elliptical trainer, but never venture over to the weights. Others, especially men, spend all of their time lifting weights (usually in a misguided quest to achieve big guns, also known as arms.) This is a good way to shortchange yourself and not develop your body to its real potential. Not only will performing a variety of exercises keep you from becoming bored, it is the only way to reach a healthy level of fitness.

In order to pick a variety of activities, you must understand the main categories of exercises. Your weekly workout plan should include a combination of Aerobic, Anaerobic, and Flexibility exercises. The next few chapters will focus on defining these types of exercises and help you understand why each is necessary.

Aerobic exercise if often referred to as "cardio training." Aerobic exercise is any activity that increases your heart rate to at least 65% of its maximum rate for an extended period of time. This type of exertion depends on oxygen from the air getting to your muscles. Your heart and lungs act together to supply that oxygen to your body, which forces them to work harder. Over time, the repetitive exertion strengthens and conditions your heart and lungs, which lowers the risk of having a heart attack. Aerobic exercise also burns fat, making it a great form of exercise for people who want to lose weight. The minute you start exercising, the amount of energy you are burning (your metabolic rate) increases to five up to 20 times what you burn when you are just sitting down! Aerobic exercise has many other immediate and long-term benefits as well. It improves your cholesterol profile, which helps lower the risk of coronary artery disease (CAD). Aerobic exercise puts positive stress on your bones, which will maintain bone strength and reduce the risk of osteoporosis. It also increases endorphins in the brain, improving your mood and sense of well being, while decreasing stress and depression. Maybe you've heard people talk about "runner's high." That's the endorphins at work!

There are many forms of aerobic exercise. Examples include jogging or brisk walking, swimming laps, cycling, roller skating, dancing, and taking a step aerobics class. You can also use cardio equipment, such as treadmills, stationary bikes, rowing machines, stair climbers, and elliptical trainers. You can pick from a variety of cardio workouts that you enjoy. If you don't enjoy your workout, the odds will be against you. Most people who begin an exercise program quit in less than a year, often because they become bored and exercise begins to feel like just another chore.

Don't make the mistake of only using a treadmill, or only taking aerobics classes. Not only will it get boring, it will take you longer to reach your fitness goals. When you perform a variety of exercises, it is called cross-training. Cross-training is important because it allows you to work various muscle groups at varying intensities, which challenges the body. For example, you might want to run one day, take a dance class another, and swim another, etc. If you enjoy exercising outdoors, mix up your routine with hiking or cross country skiing. However, don't worry too much about balancing various forms of aerobic activity at first. The most important thing is that you just pick something that you can do and get off your butt and start moving! If all else fails, go for a brisk walk.

Target Heart Rate: To determine if you are working aerobically, you need to figure out your target heart rate, which begins by knowing your maximum heart rate. Generally, the further you are from your maximum heart rate during moderate aerobic activity, the fitter you are. The most accurate way of determining your personal maximum heart rate is to have it tested by a healthcare provider using a treadmill stress test. You can also get a general idea by simply using an age-adjusted formula. To do this, subtract your age from 220. Now multiply your maximum heart rate by .6 and .8. This is the target zone that you want to stay in during aerobic exercise.

Calculating Max Heart Rate

Here's an example using a 45 year old:

Maximum Heart Rate: 175 (220 − 45 = 175)

Target Zone Heart Rate: 105 to 140 (220 x .6 = 105, 220 x .8 = 140)

You can check to see if you are in your target zone by taking your pulse at least once during your workout. Check your pulse while you are still moving. If you need to slow down your activity to feel your pulse, try to at least keep walking or marching in place. You can also buy a heart-rate monitor to check your pulse. They cost around $50 for a basic model.

Another way to check your pulse is by using your Carotid artery or the inside of your wrist. The Carotid artery is found by touching your Adam's apple. Reach two fingers toward the side of your neck, where you will feel the muscles that run from your collar bone to the base of your head. Your pulse is just in front of these muscles, about four fingers widths from the Adam's apple. Now, take your index and middle fingers, and lightly feel the pulse. Don't use your thumb, because you may feel your thumb's pulse and be confused. Also, do not press on your neck! Detecting your pulse only requires a light touch and pushing too hard on your Carotid artery can be dangerous. Count the number of beats in a ten second period and then multiply by six, or count for fifteen seconds and multiply by four. Either way will give you the number of heart beats per minute.

So, if the 45 year-old male in our example counted his pulse during a walk and determined his heart rate was 100 beats per minute, he would want to pick up the pace in order to be in his target zone. If his pulse was 160 beats per minute, he would want to slow down. The goal in aerobic exercise is to challenge your heart, but not to overtax it. Within two months of starting an exercise routine, you should be able to increase the intensity of your workouts by using your heart rate as a guide. (Note: Some medications, including beta blockers for blood pressure control, make it impossible to use your pulse as a way of judging how hard you are working. If you are unsure about how your medication will affect your workouts, consult your doctor.)

The Talk Test: You can also use your breathing as a loose indicator of aerobic exercise. Your breathing should be faster, but you should not feel out of breath or feel like it is hard to breath. If you can carry on a normal conversation, you are not working hard enough... pick up the pace! On the flip side, if you can't talk at all you're working too hard and are experiencing oxygen deficit. This means you have moved into anaerobic exercise and are no longer using oxygen to burn fat. Remember the goal is to burn fat!

How Often: For best results, schedule some form of aerobic exercise 3-6 times per week for a duration of 30 minutes. When you are first starting to exercise, just do as much as you can until your stamina builds. If you can only handle 10 minutes, that's fine. Keep working on it and eventually you should be able to maintain an aerobic heart rate for 20-30 minutes. New research has also shown that interval training can be very beneficial for burning fat in a short period of time. Plus it will make your time fly by while exercising. Intervals are simply time segments between work and recovery. The best ratio should be 2 to 1 (2 parts recovery to 1 part work). You may want to start with 15 second work followed by 30 second recovery until you can work up to a minute work to two minute recovery. During the work phase increase your intensity whether that be speed, resistance or incline, and during your recovery bring your heart rate back down. You can build from there. However, if you start exercising and feel you must quit, do not stop moving right away. It is important that you cool-down (more on proper cool-downs later.) If you feel that you can't fit in 30 minutes of aerobic exercise, try to squeeze in a few 10 minute sessions during the day. New research shows that you will still enjoy the benefits of a cardiovascular workout even with multiple, shorter workouts.

Most importantly, enjoy your aerobic exercise. It is a wonderful way to feel energized, alive, and empowered. With every step, stroke, or row, you are taking control of your health and moving your body in the right direction.

BUTT KICKIN': For an exercise to be an aerobic activity, it must increase your heart rate by using major muscle groups for an extended period of time. There are many benefits to regular aerobic exercise, including strengthening your heart, losing weight, and boosting your mood. You can, and should, partake in various types of aerobic exercise into your routine. Some of the many forms include walking, bicycling, dancing, and using a piece of cardio equipment. Try to incorporate 30 minutes of aerobic exercise at least 3 to 6 days per week.

My Favorite Cardiovascular Activities:

❑ walking   ❑ jogging   ❑ swimming

❑ cycling   ❑ roller blading   ❑ dancing

❑ aerobics classes ❑ rowing   ❑ _____

WALKING

Walking is a great form of aerobic exercise. It gets its own special section in this book, because it is one of the best ways for the true beginner to start feeling and seeing results. Walking is easy, safe, and free (unless you count the cost of your shoes.) It also is one of the simplest exercises to fit into your busy lifestyle.

Research has shown that taking 10,000 steps a day can bring you a host of physical benefits, including reducing your risk of heart disease, preventing some cancers, and lowering your blood pressure. Yet, most Americans don't even come close. The average person walks only 900 to 3,000 steps a day! 10,000 steps is generally between four and five miles, depending on your stride. Most of us can cover that distance in about an hour if we move briskly, but you don't have to take all of those steps at once.

Perhaps you want to start with a 30-minute walk before and after work. You can also break it down by simply moving more throughout the day. Unless you live in a city, you may not be able to walk to work or to the store, but you can find ways to walk more. Most Americans are overly dependent on their cars. Stop wasting time circling parking lots. There are always spaces available at the end of the lot furthest from the mall. Park there and walk. Take the stairs whenever possible. Give up one half hour of television, basically *Get Off Your Butt and Do Something*. Ask your partner to take an evening walk with you. You'll both get some exercise while enjoying valuable time together. Although walking alone will not bring all of the benefits of a well-rounded fitness program, it is a great start. Empower yourself and be creative. You will be able to find all kinds of ways to include walking in your daily routine.

THE SCIENCE BEHIND AEROBIC EXERCISE

If you have read the previous chapter on aerobic exercise, you already have enough information to get started. This chapter is not a "How to..." It's a "Why?" So, if you're interested in what is going on inside your body as you workout, enjoy the following explanation. If you simply want the facts necessary to begin your workouts, jump ahead to the next chapter, *Anaerobic Exercise & Strength Training*.

As soon as you start exercising, incredible functions within your body kick-in and go to work. Your body's first priority is getting the energy necessary to allow you to move. During the first three minutes of aerobic exercise, you really are not exercising aerobically at all. Instead, your muscles are intent on burning glycogen, which is a sugar that your muscles store for quick energy. At this point, your muscles are working anaerobically, meaning without oxygen. As your body starts to work, it is common to feel a burning sensation in your muscles. This is lactic acid released during anaerobic exercise. Lactic acid is created as your body burns its glycogen. Don't worry, as you move into the aerobic part of your workout, this feeling will fade as blood starts bringing oxygen to your muscles. That oxygen will help burn the glycogen and will stop the production of lactic acid.

It will usually take about 20 minutes to burn all of your glycogen. When the glycogen is used up, the body will begin burning the fat it has stored in an effort to produce more glycogen. As long as you stay within your target heart rate and keep getting oxygen to the muscles, the longer you exercise, the more body fat you will burn. After you stop exercising, you body must replace the glycogen it has used, so it relies on fatty tissue to produce more. This fat burning process can last for 24 to 48 hours after you stop exercising, that's pretty awesome!

ANAEROBIC EXERCISE AND STRENGTH TRAINING

Anaerobic exercise is crucial for gaining muscle and building strength. It can also aid in weight loss by increasing your metabolism (the number of calories you burn in a day.) Anaerobic activity boosts your heart rate up to 80 – 90% of your maximum heart rate during very intense, but short, bursts of exertion, which are followed by a period of rest. Anaerobic means "without oxygen" or "without air." During anaerobic exercise, oxygen from the lungs does not have time to travel to the muscles. Weight training and sprinting are forms of anaerobic exercise. Longer activities, like boxing and football are also classified as anaerobic because the periods of exertion are very intense, but brief.

Unlike aerobic exercise, which strengthens the heart and lungs by moving large muscles thousands of times against gravity, strength training provides so much resistance that it only takes relatively few repetitions to reap major benefits. Some people think that strength training is only for body builders or those overly concerned with their appearance. While it is true that many people strength train because they want a nice, toned physique, strength training is for everyone, even the elderly.

There are many reasons to strength train. First and foremost, it is the only type of exercise that can slow, and even reverse, the aging process. Working against resistance can reduce your risk of developing heart disease, osteoporosis, and diabetes. It has also been shown to fight various types of chronic pain, including arthritis. You will also become stronger, which will make all types of daily activities, like carrying groceries or children, easier. For example, the average golfer who strength trains has significantly more driving power than those who do not exercise regularly.

In just a couple of months of strength training, you are also likely to notice an increase in your endurance. Think about how it feels when you do a set of intense squats. That "burn" you feel is a by-product of anaerobic activity, called lactic acid. Lactic acid makes your muscles tired. It must be burned up by the body during a period of rest before the exercise can be resumed. The rest, or recovery, period also allows the muscles to receive oxygen, which is needed to restore energy. Over time, you will gain endurance and higher lactic acid tolerance ability, meaning it will take longer to become fatigued.

In order to gain strength, you have to give the muscle more stimulation than it is used to. There are many different strength training exercises, such as free weights, selectorized machines, stretch tubing and bands, and a thousand other pieces of equipment. Many anaerobic exercises, like squats, pushups or lunges, do not require any equipment.

If you are new to working out, it is important to understand how to correctly perform at least one (but ideally, several) strength training exercises for each of your major muscle groups. It is recommended that you hire a fitness professional for at least a few sessions. If you don't feel comfortable hiring a fitness professional, ask a knowledgeable friend to help you, or attend a body sculpting class (these are standard classes at most gyms.) Some people also like to learn from books or videos. However, a conscious decision was made to not include specific instructions on strength training exercises in this book, because it is always a good idea to have a live person help you at first. Even if you think you understand the pictures or instructions in a book, beginners are likely to perform at least some of the exercises incorrectly. Improperly performing exercises will waste time by not allowing you to get the most out of your workout and can lead to injury. Below is a list of your major muscle groups and a few basic, corresponding exercises that will be easy to have someone teach you. Keep in mind, there are countless exercises that you can learn and you will eventually want to incorporate a variety of exercises into your strength training routine.

The Muscle Groups

Lower Body Major Muscle Groups:

Quadriceps (Quads): This is the large group of muscles on the front part of your leg that run from your hips to your knees. Squats and leg presses will benefit your quadriceps, as will lunges and leg extensions.

Hamstrings: This muscle group is the opposite to the quadriceps, and is located along the back of your leg, from below your buttocks to above your knees. The quadriceps exercises listed above will also tone the hamstrings. Deadlifts and Leg curls are designed to target the hamstrings.

Gluteals: This is the group of muscles, including the gluteus maximus, which make up your buttocks. Squats, Stair Steps and leg presses are common exercises for the gluteals.

Hip abductors and adductors: These are the smaller group of muscles that form your inner and outer thigh. The abductors are on the outside of your thigh and help your leg move away from your body. The adductors create your inner thigh. There are a lot of exercises for this muscle group, including side lying leg lifts, hip machines, and standing cable pulls.

Calf: Your calf muscles are under your knee and form the back of the lower leg. They are formed by the gastrocnemius muscle, which gives the calf its round shape, and the soleus, which is a flat muscle that is located under the gastrocnemius. Many of the lower body exercises you perform will also benefit the calf muscles. However, to target your gastrocnemius muscle, you can do standing calf raises. Seated calf machines and bent knee raises will mostly strengthen your soleus.

Upper Body Major Muscle Groups:

Deltoids (Shoulders): The deltoid muscles form your shoulders. They are comprised of three different parts, the front deltoid (anterior), the middle deltoid (medial) and the rear deltoid (posterior). You'll want to incorporate a variety of deltoid exercises into your workouts to strengthen each of these muscles. Rear, front, and lateral raises performed with light dumbbells are simple, but very effective. Push-ups are also great for your shoulders.

Biceps: This is the muscle a lot of guys (and some women) love to flex and show-off (also known as "The Gun Show". This is the front of your upper arm. The best move is a basic bicep curl. You can do this with dumbbells, barbells, or a machine.

Triceps: This is the opposing muscle group to the bicep. The triceps are located on the back of your upper arm. A major concern of most women is to keep the triceps from sagging, that's when they are called "Nana Arms", and "Bat Wings". Exercises for the triceps include kick-backs, dips and overhead presses.

Pectoralis Major (Pecs): You often hear people refer to this muscle as the "pecs." It is a large, fan shaped muscle that covers the upper chest. Pushups, bench presses, and pec machines are some of the exercises that will benefit this area.

Trapezius (Traps): This is the upper area of your back, also called your "traps." Upright rows or weighted shoulder shrugs will target your trapezius muscle.

Rhomboids: The rhomboids are in the middle of your upper back, between your shoulder blades. You can work this group with chin-ups, bent over rows, seated rows and other resistance moves that bring the shoulder blades together.

Latisimus Dorsi (Lats): These are the largest muscles of your back. Toned and strong lats give your back a V shape, and make your waist look smaller. You can strengthen this area by using a pull-down machine or doing pull-ups and one arm bent over rows.

Low Back: Many people suffer from a weak lower back. Toning this area will help maintain good posture and alleviate low-back pain. Studies have consistently shown that strength training is an effective way to reduce or even eliminate low back pain. You can use a back extension machine, or perform simple back extension exercises without a machine.

Abdominals: This group of muscles, often called "abs", include the rectus abdominus, which runs the length of your abdomen, and the external obliques, which form the front and sides off your abdomen. Strong abdominals help support the lower back. There are many great exercises to strengthen this area, including the standard crunch, reverse curls, and plank positions.

BUTT KICKIN': List one exercise per muscle group:

Quad: _____

Hamstring: _____

Glutes: _____

Hips: _____

Calves: _____

Delts: _____

Biceps: _____

Triceps: _____

Traps: _____

Rhomboids:_____

Lats:_____

Low Back: _____

Abdominals: _____

Check out the resource section of www.GetOffYourButtNDoSomething.com for video demonstrations of many of these exercises.

Exercise Order

It is strongly recommended that you have someone show you how to perform some, or all of these exercises, even if that instruction comes during a group strength training class. Until then, to achieve the best results possible, you should train your larger muscle groups first and/or perform exercises that utilize several muscle groups before working the smaller groups. By working out this way, you can attempt the most demanding exercises when you are not fatigued. For instance, push-ups are quite demanding and require the strength of several muscle groups. You'll be able to complete more of them if you have not fatigued yourself with tricep-kickbacks. Although there are many ideas about the ultimate routine, beginners can benefit from working out muscle groups in the following order, choose one exercise per body part for a full body workout:

1. Legs

2. Chest

3. Back

4. Shoulders

5. Arms

6. Abs and low back

Sets and Reps

People new to fitness are sometimes confused by the terms "reps" and "sets." A set means that you are repeating the same exercise a number of times without resting. Repetitions or "reps" are simply the number of times you perform the exercise in the set. For example, lifting and lowering the weight during a bicep curl counts as one rep. So if you want to do three sets of ten reps, you would lift and lower the weight ten times in a row without stopping, rest for a moment, then repeat that sequence two more times. Generally, a person new to strength training should rest for at least one minute between sets.

Speed

Do not rush when performing strength training exercises. Try to take one or two seconds to lift the weight and three to four seconds to lower it during each rep. If you go too fast, momentum will be propelling the weight, not your muscle. Movements that are too fast may cause unnecessary strain and injury. You also want to concentrate on achieving a full range of motion, meaning that each exercise should involve the full range of the joint in a single, controlled movement. The repetition should strengthen your muscle by contracting, while stretching the opposing muscle. Sometimes you will see someone at the gym lifting heavy weights by jerking or throwing them up to contract the muscle. This is improper form. If you have to jerk the weight up to contract the muscle, the weight is too heavy for you. The amount of weight you lift is less important than lifting it correctly. Think quality over quantity.

How Much Weight

Start with a weight that allows you to complete at least 12-15 repetitions using proper form. By the time you finish the set, you should be fatigued. Once you can complete 15 repetitions in a set, increase the amount of weight by 5%. Now, you will no longer be able to complete 15 reps, so just aim for 10 – 12 reps. When this weight becomes less challenging at 12 reps, increase it by 5% again. Five percent is just a guideline. You can experiment with other increments; just don't increase the weight by more than 10% at any time. Over time, this alternate progression of increasing weight and then building on the number of repetitions in each set will help you gain strong, toned muscles.

Muscle Soreness vs. Pain

A day or two after lifting weights, it is common to feel some soreness. Physiologists believe that stress placed on muscles during strength training can result in small tears. This may cause some delayed onset muscle soreness (DOMS), but as the tissue heals, the muscle will increase in size and strength. It is also important to realize that the body is burning calories while repairing the muscles. This is the "after-burn" effect from resistance training that you won't get from cardio alone.

Forget that old saying "no pain, no gain" when you are working out. You are better off thinking, "better safe than sorry." You should feel fatigued after a set, but you should not feel real pain. If you ever feel joint pain, nerve pain, or a sudden, intense strain, it is time to ease up. Don't ever push yourself to the point of pain because you will likely end up with an injury. Muscle tears, strains, and sprains can take a long time to heal, which could mean months of forced inactivity and the feeling of failure.

How Often

You should ideally schedule some form of strength training for at least 30 minutes, two to three times a week, but not on consecutive days. Your muscles need time to recover after a strength training workout. For this reason, it is important to wait at least 48 hours before scheduling another session. For example, if you strength train your whole body on Monday, you can do an aerobic workout on Tuesday, and more strength training on Wednesday. Alternately, you could work out only your upper body on Monday and focus on strengthening the lower body on Tuesday. Either way is fine; just don't train the same muscle groups back-to-back.

Women and Weights

One of the biggest myths surrounding strength training is that it will make women bulk-up. It's a myth that was debunked in the first part of this book, but it is such a pervasive misconception, that it bears repeating: WOMEN WILL NOT BULK-UP! Compared to men, women don't gain a lot of size from lifting weights because they have up to 30 times less of the hormones that stimulate muscle growth. Study after study has proven that women who strength train on a regular basis are leaner, not bigger. That's because women typically lose much more fat though anaerobic exercise than they will gain in muscle. In one large-scale study, women who strength trained at least two times a week for two months gained about 1 ½ pounds of lean muscle mass, but lost 3 ½ pounds of fat! As your body gains muscle from strength training, your resting metabolism is increased. That means, even when you are sitting on the couch watching TV, you'll be burning more calories than people who do not strength train! Every pound of muscle you gain will burn nearly 35 extra calories a day.

BUTT KICKIN': When strength training, it is important to perform exercises that challenge each of the main muscle groups. In order to ensure proper form and safety, it is always a good idea to have someone show you how to correctly perform new exercises. Strength training should be done for a minimum of 30 minutes, 2 to 3 times a week, but not on consecutive days.

Days I'm going to Strength Train are:

_____   _____   _____

THE SPOT REDUCING MYTH

Spot reducing means getting rid of fat in just one area of your body through some sort of anaerobic exercise. For instance, you've seen the infomercials that claim using a certain gadget will give you six-pack abs or a smaller butt. Some women will do hundreds of leg-lifts trying to get rid of saddlebags. Men who have "beer bellies" may do a lot of crunches. These products and exercise habits will set up you for failure. While any exercise may help you build muscle in a particular area of your body, nothing will remove fat from only one part of your body.

Your muscles rest under a layer of fat. If they are covered with too much fat, you will look flabby or appear to have cellulite. The only way to reduce that layer is to slowly lose fat over your entire body through aerobic exercise. As the fat is burned off, the muscle that you built through toning exercises will become more apparent.

Unfortunately, you may not lose fat in your trouble spots first, even if you are working really hard toward your goals. Where you will lose fat depends largely on your genetic makeup. However, with a consistent regimen of cardio, strength training and proper nutrition you will see improvements.

BUTT KICKIN': Trying to reduce fat on just one body part *never* works. If you want to tone a specific area of your body, combine aerobic exercise and strength training exercises. Keep doing those sit-ups and leg lifts. Just make sure that they are only one component of a comprehensive program that works your entire body.

Body Parts I want to Strength and Tone:

1. _____

2. _____

3. _____

WARMING UP AND COOLING DOWN

Every time you workout, it is important to properly warm-up and cool down. Many times people skip the warm-up and cool down because they are in a rush to get through their workout. However, it is very important to realize that a proper warm-up and cool down are essential parts of the workout.

Warm-Up

A gentle warm-up prepares your body for the work to come. When you warm-up, you increase the temperature of your muscles, which increases your flexibility, improving your range of motion and reducing the chance of injury. During your warm-up, your blood vessels will dilate slowly, which lessens the stress on the heart.

Start each workout with a 5 to 10 minute warm-up that consists of low-impact, easy aerobic exercise. Walking, marching in place, or mild intensity aerobic dance all work well. If you are warming up for an aerobic workout, you can simply perform the exercise at a lower speed. For instance, if you want to spend 30 minutes on a stationary bike, pedal slowly with no resistance to warm-up, and then gradually begin to increase the intensity until you reach your target heart rate. The warm-up can count as part of the time you spend working out. After your warm-up, stretch the muscles you have just used. For instance, after warming up on a stationary bike, you will want to stretch your quadriceps, hamstrings, calves, and glutes (your butt).

Even when warming up for an anaerobic workout, you still want to do at least five minutes of a gentle aerobic exercise. This is called a "general" warm-up, because it does not target any specific body part. After your general warm-up, it is recommended that you perform a "specific" warm-up. A specific warm-up is a light set of an exercise that targets the muscle group you will be working. The specific warm-up should be done as the first exercise for each muscle group. For example, if you are going to work your lower body with leg presses, you might first want to warm-up your quadriceps, hamstrings and glutes by doing a set of squats while holding no weight. If you are going to be doing chest presses, do one warm-up set using very light weights before getting on with the more butt kicking work.

Although stretching can be a good way to help your body prepare for the work ahead, never stretch before completing a general warm-up. This is very important because stretching when your muscles are cold can increase the chance of injury. Perform only static stretching. Never bounce. Also, continue to breathe. Holding your breath can cause your blood pressure to spike. Warm up stretches should be very gentle and should not hurt or provide an uncomfortable straining sensation. Hold each stretch for at least five seconds.

Now that you are warmed up, start working out. Never allow more than a few minutes to pass between the completion of your warm-up and your main exercise.

Cool Down

After you have completed your exercises, it is crucial that you cool down. If you simply stop, you can suddenly reduce your blood pressure, which can be dangerous for some people. Cooling down can also help in the body's recovery process and reduce muscle soreness. Researchers have discovered that a cool down can reduce lactic acid levels faster than by simply stopping. The cool down can be as simple as slowly walking around a room, or slowing down your aerobic exercise. Like warm-ups, cool downs should last for about 5 to 10 minutes. Ideally, you want to gradually bring your heart rate to only about 10 to 15 beats above its resting rate.

Finally, stretch the muscles that you have used. Your muscles will be very warm now, so the cool down stretches should last longer than the warm up stretches. Hold each for about 20-30 seconds. Again, don't bounce. You want nice, long static stretches. This should feel good or only give you mild discomfort. If you experience pain, you've gone too far.

FLEXIBILITY TRAINING

Ask someone about their workout and they may tell you how far they run or how much weight they lift, but very few people will mention flexibility training. Stretching before or after a workout is the first thing people skip when they feel pressed for time. However, this means they are missing out on a major component of true physical fitness. Think of fitness as a triangle. One side is aerobic activity, one side is strength training, and one side is flexibility. You don't want to neglect flexibility training any more than you want to give up your aerobic and anaerobic workouts. They are all essential to a well-rounded exercise routine.

In layman's terms, flexibility is how far your body can comfortably reach, twist, or bend. Increasing your flexibility will help you in nearly every physical activity throughout the day, from reaching up to grab something, to bending down to tie your shoes. Flexibility may help with coordination, making you less likely to fall. It also allows your joints to experience their full range of motion. Limber joints will allow you to be active and limber as you age and you'll have less of a chance of becoming injured.

Becoming more flexible may mean the end of some types of chronic pain. Tight muscles cause pain in unexpected places. For instance, lower back pain is an extremely common problem among adults. Did you know that it can occur because of tight muscles in your hips? When you sit all day, your hip flexors tighten, yet your gluteal muscles become loose. Now you have an imbalance in which some joints and bones are stressing under too much weight. The next thing you know, your hamstrings tighten up, your pelvis gets out of line, and your back hurts. Instead of reaching for pain medicine, you should probably just correct your body's imbalances by stretching.

Stretching also feels good. Once you get into the habit of stretching, you won't feel the same on days you skip your flexibility exercises. When you experience how much better a limber body feels, chances are you'll be hooked. You just need to make it a habit in order to enjoy its full benefits.

When you are stretching, keep the following in mind:

- No Bouncing! I've mentioned this already, but it is very important. Bouncing can make the muscle go too far and it will increase your chances of injury.

- Stretch each of your major muscle groups at least once, preferably twice or more.

- Hold each stretch for at least 20 seconds or more.

- Breathe throughout the stretch. Start by inhaling, as you exhale begin the stretch. Continue to take deep breaths. Inhale as you leave the stretch.

- Extend only to the point of tension, not pain.

- When you are trying to stretch the back, try to keep the low back against the floor or mat. Work only the muscles required to change position. In many cases, this will be the abdomen.

When to Stretch

Incorporating stretching into your exercise plan does not have to be complicated. Every time you workout, either aerobically or anaerobically, you should stretch as part of your cool-down. Stretching can also be very helpful when done between strength training sets. Instead of just resting during the recovery period, stretch the muscles you have been working. You will find that the next set often feels easier. Many experts believe you will experience more strength gains if you stretch immediately following anaerobic exercise. You can experience even greater benefits by making flexibility training the focus of a workout, thanks to the increasing popularity of yoga, tai chi, and Pilates.

How Often

You should try to stretch as part of each workout. Ideally, you want to spend a minimum of 30 minutes stretching each week. However, this is the least amount you want to do. By stretching more, you will reap the benefits of increased flexibility.

BUTT KICKIN': The muscles I need to stretch the most are:
_____. I plan on stretching ____ times per week.

OTHER BUTT KICKIN' METHODS WORTH CHECKING OUT

Now that you understand the basic principles behind aerobic, anaerobic, and flexibility exercises, you can start exploring subcategories of exercising. There are many different methods of working out that will not only keep you from getting bored with your routine, but will give you another way to firm, tone, and lengthen your muscles.

Circuit Training

Circuit training is a great way to maximize your efforts in a minimal amount of time. During a circuit training workout, you perform a series of short exercises back-to-back, without stopping. Because your heart rate stays elevated throughout the workout, you can burn a lot of calories while strengthening your heart and muscles. Although you can just do all strength training or all cardio exercises, combining a few of each will provide added benefits. This type of circuit training keeps workouts from getting boring and is very efficient. Because circuit training is tailored to the individual, it works well for people of all fitness levels.

When designing your circuit training routine, allow at least 5 to 10 minutes to both warm up and cool down. Your circuit should last at least 20 minutes, but not much more than 40 minutes. You can do a quick full-body workout, trying to complete one exercise for each major muscle group, or break up your circuit training into sessions for upper and lower body. For example a lower body circuit might consist of 3 minutes of step aerobics, 1 minute of squats, back to step aerobics, 1 minute of alternating lunges, 1 minute of jumping rope, followed by 1 minute of standing leg lifts (30 seconds on each side). After completing the full circuit, repeat it enough times until you have performed the desired number of sets of each exercise. To get the maximum benefits in compact circuit training workouts, it is a good idea to focus on compound movements instead of using weight machines.

Compound movements engage more than one muscle group. For example, squats are considered a compound movement because they primarily work your thighs and glutes, but also strengthen your calves and lower back.

Remember, just like in all strength training, the muscles you work will need time to rest. Circuit training on consecutive days is fine. Just don't work the same body parts on back-to-back days.

Many boot camp programs are designed around doing circuits. They can also be a lot of fun since there are others going through the same program and are led by a qualified trainer.

Interval Training

After you have been training for six to eight weeks, you may be ready to pump up the intensity of your cardio routines with an interval program. During an interval training workout, you go between intense bursts of speed and slower, recovery periods. You repeat this cycle several times during a workout. A very simple interval workout can be achieved by walking on a treadmill. Let's say that you normally walk on the treadmill at 3.7MPH for 20 minutes (not counting warm-up and cool down.). During interval training you may walk at 3.7MPH for 3 minutes and then walk for 4.2MPH for 1 minute. Repeat this sequence until you have exercised for 20 minutes.

As soon as you try this method, you will discover that interval training is much more taxing than the sustained pace cardio you may be used to. During the brief bursts, you want to try to get your target heart rate to about 75% maximum. This is intense, but only lasts for a short period of time. At first, you may only be able to do one or two intervals per workout. Just keeping working at it. Intervals are a great way to build your cardiovascular endurance. Any form of cardio exercise can be turned into an interval workout by simply using your target heart rate as a guide or relying on your perceived level of exertion.

Below is a sample of a 20 minute, intense routine using perceived exertion. On a scale of 1 to 10, 1 requires almost no exertion and 10 is the very most energy you can expend. If attempting this workout, remember to begin and end with a warm-up and cool down (refer to the previous section on warm-ups and cool downs.) You can increase your perceived level of exertion on cardio equipment by increasing the pace, and/or resistance of the machine.

INTERVAL TRAINING WORKOUT
(AFTER WARMING UP)

To identify your exertion level, use the "talk test". If you can carry on a normal conversation while exercising your exertion level is between 1 and 5. If you find it difficult to carry on a conversation and must take a breath after every sentence than you are at a level 7, if you are spitting out words your level is 9, and if you can't speak at all (which also means you can't breathe) you are at a level 10. You should never get to level 10.

Using the above reference I want you to warm up for five minutes at a level 5. Then for the next 4 minutes I want you to increase your effort level by one step each minute. For example, minute 6 will be at your exertion level 6, minute 7 at exertion level 7 and so on until you reach exertion level 9. After that minute, drop back down to exertion level 6 and repeat that climb to exertion level 9 at one minute intervals. You should work your way up to completing three peaks followed by a three minute cool down at exertion level 5. Graphically it would look like the following.

TIME	Level 5	Level 6	Level 7	Level 8	Level 9
1 – 5 Minutes	■				
Minute 6	■	■			
Minute 7	■	■	■		
Minute 8	■	■	■	■	
Minute 9	■	■	■	■	■
Minute 10	■	■			
Minute 11	■	■	■		
Minute 12	■	■	■	■	
Minute 13	■	■	■	■	■
Minute 14	■	■			
Minute 15	■	■	■		
Minute 16	■	■	■	■	
Minute 17	■	■	■	■	■
Minute 18	■				
Minute 19	■				
Minute 20	■				

Split Routines

As a beginner, you might want to strength train all of your major muscle groups in one session. Full body workouts can be very effective, especially if you are pressed for time during the week. However, as your workouts progress, you may want to consider split routines. During split routines, you work on just a few body parts, but hit them with more types of exercises and sets. You may also use heavier weights. The next day, you work different body parts.

There are several ways to split your routine. You may try one method for a few weeks and then decide to mix it up a bit. The most basic split routine involves dividing your workout into upper and lower body. For instance, on Mondays and Thursdays work your upper body. Tuesdays and Fridays could be reserved for legs.

Another great way to hit your entire body during the week is to split your program into push and pull exercises. Pushing exercises can include squats, bench press, triceps kickbacks, and lateral raises (plus, many, many more.) Pushing motions usually involve quadriceps, chest, triceps and shoulders. A pull routine will most often work the hamstrings, back, sometimes the shoulders, and biceps. These exercises can include leg curls, lat pull downs, upright rows and bicep curls. Many abdominal exercises, like crunches, also fall into the pulling category.

Push/pull routines imitate the movements your body must perform during daily tasks. This is important for every age group, especially the elderly. For example, an older person might find getting out of a chair increasingly difficult. A pushing exercise like tricep dips mimics the same action necessary to rise from a seated position. Strengthening in this way makes functioning in everyday life easier and more enjoyable.

Another split routine could involve only strength training one or two muscle groups per day. This is a good way to open up more time for cardio. However, if you plan to do this, remember to increase the number of exercises you do for each body part. Pick at least three exercises for each muscle group.

Core Training

Core training is very popular in gyms these days. But, don't mistake this as just another fad. Core training targets your trunk, including your abdominal area, lower back, and the upper part of your hips. The main focus of core training is the deep muscles of the torso that attach to the spine, pelvis, and shoulders. To feel this group of muscles, sit up straight and try to squeeze your belly button to the back of your spine.

A strong core is going to give you a nice, flat stomach (providing the muscles aren't covered by a thick layer of fat.) Core training is about much more than looking great. This is true functional fitness, meaning that it helps you maintain the muscles that are necessary for everyday living. You rely on your core almost every time you move your body. A stable core can help correct postural imbalances, reducing the chance of injury. It will also improve muscle strength, endurance, and flexibility. Some studies show that it even helps increase bone density.

Core training is an entirely different approach than strength training. In strength training, you focus on the movement of single or multiple joints to work against resistance. In core training, no single muscle is isolated. Instead, all of the deep muscles of the trunk are activated at the same time.

Although standard crunches and push-ups could be considered core work, there are many new, exciting training techniques. Some of the most popular core training methods include Pilates, stability ball movements, and exercises with medicine balls. Core training group classes at gyms often combine many different techniques, including yoga and tai chi inspired moves. During most of the classes, instructors encourage students to squeeze their belly button to their spine, as described above. This is called abdominal bracing.

Because core training relies on a person's own body weight and is easily adapted to any fitness level, classes are proving to be very popular among all ages and genders. There are also many core training fitness videos now available for home use.

Mind/Body Exercises

Nothing in recent times has swept the fitness industry like the enormous popularity of mind/body exercises. Although many types of mind/body exercises have influenced core training, these are individual, separate types of exercise. Mind/Body exercise means many different things. Some people perform these disciplines as a way to reduce stress or experience a spiritual connection. Others just see mind/body exercises as another demanding form of exercise that can produce fantastic physical results. Either way, the most popular mind/body exercise forms in the United States are Yoga and Pilates. Other workouts include Tai chi, the Alexander Technique and Feldenkrais.

Yoga originated from India and has been performed for thousands of years. The word "yoga" is a Sanskrit term for "union." Some classes, especially at yoga studios, focus on mediation and spirituality. However, many yoga classes have dispensed with these elements and have become strictly athletic workouts. There are many forms of yoga. Two of the most popular ones offered at health clubs are Hatha yoga, which focuses on posture and breathing, and Astanga yoga. Astanga yoga is also known as "power yoga" and provides an intense workout that stretches and strengthens the body while relieving stress and improving balance. Yoga can work you very hard and then leave you feeling energized, so it is no wonder people often talk about it as giving them a natural high.

Despite the misconception that you have to be very flexible, or "new age," to take a yoga class, almost anyone can benefit from yoga. When taking a class for the first time, make sure you work at your own pace. Yoga is meant to be an individual practice, so don't feel competitive or intimidated by the person next to you that can bend like a circus contortionist.

Pilates is named after its developer, Joseph Pilates. He created the exercise to help dancers recover from injuries and build strength. There are two forms of Pilates. One is completed on a mat, usually in a class setting, or you can take lessons on Pilates Reformer machines. Both forms focus almost exclusively on you buttocks, abs, lower back, and thighs. Like the core training moves it helped inspire, Pilates requires you to engage many muscles at once. Pilates and Yoga are unique forms of exercise in that you practice them, not master them. Just when you think you've got it, there's another slightly harder way to perform an exercise or hold a posture.

Group Pilates classes and yoga only require a mat and comfortable clothing. Because these types of exercise can be demanding, you can perform a mind/body exercise in place of one or two regularly scheduled flexibility or strength training sessions per week.

EVERY TIME YOU EXERCISE

No matter what form of exercise you plan on doing, there are a few, basic safety precautions that apply.

Start every new type of exercise slowly. Eventually, you will be able to increase duration and intensity. If you do too much right away, you may injure yourself. Err on the side of caution, especially if you have not worked out in a while.

Drink water before, during, and after a workout. It is imperative that you stay hydrated. Try to drink 8 to 16 ounces in the two hours before you workout. Then during your training session, try to drink a half-cup for every 20 minutes you workout. After working out, drink even more water. Experts recommend that you drink two cups of fluid for every pound of body weight you lose during exercise.

Don't eat a full meal for about two hours before exercising. You may need a small snack before an intense workout just so you have enough energy to make it through the workout.

Don't hold your breath. This is a common mistake. Always focus on steady breathing that includes exhaling while your muscles are contracting and inhaling when you are coming out of a movement. For example, breathe out as a weight is lifted and in as it is lowered.

Generally, you want to bend from the hips, not the waist (unless you are doing certain flexibility exercises.) Try to keep your back straight.

Listen to your body. If you feel like you are not getting enough out of your routine, increase the intensity. Your body will also warn you if you start to do too much. If you feel pain, stop! If you experience chest pain, irregular heartbeat, nausea, light-headedness, or extreme fatigue, seek immediate medical attention.

BUILDING YOUR WEEKLY ROUTINE

It doesn't matter when you start your workout week. Some people like to start a new week on Sunday or Monday, while others pick another day that best fits their schedule. No matter when your weekly program begins, you should take a few minutes at the start of each cycle to create a plan of attack for the upcoming week. When you are writing out your workout routine, think about what worked the previous week and what may need to be rearranged. Then, post your schedule where you see it every day. Every time you complete a workout, put a checkmark beside it or cross it off. Occasionally, something will happen and you will have to skip a workout midweek. If that happens, plan to complete that workout on one of your days off. If you still can't fit it in, just make a note of it and try to meet all of your goals next week.

BUTT KICKIN': Determine the days and times you will be working out on a weekly basis and mark it in your calendar as an appointment. You are less likely to skip it if it is scheduled.

Monday   ___   AM/PM

Tuesday   ___   AM/PM

Wednesday   ___   AM/PM

Thursday   ___   AM/PM

Friday   ___   AM/PM

Saturday   ___   AM/PM

Sunday   ___   AM/PM

BEGINNER'S BASIC WORKOUT

Here is a sample workout plan that is perfect for beginners. It is a five or six day program that incorporates aerobic, anaerobic and flexibility conditioning, along with an optional workout. Use the recommended exercises in the *Anaerobic Exercise* section for the strength workouts. For cardio, try to do a few different activities each week. Anything is fine as long as it gets you to your target heart rate. For each workout, remember to include a warm-up and a cool down, plus stretching time for flexibility.

Monday	Full Body Strength training (Upper/Lower body and abs)
Tuesday	30 – 40 minutes Cardio
Wednesday	30- 40 minutes Cardio
Thursday	Full Body Strength Training (Upper/Lower body and abs
Friday	Day off, yoga, or take a long walk
Saturday	30-40 minutes Cardio + core workout
Sunday	Day off

Beginner's Split Routine

After you have worked out using the beginner's routine for a while, try to mix things up with this split routine. Follow the routine shown below, but feel free to try various combinations of exercises. Just remember not to work the same muscle groups on consecutive days. Each workout should include a warm-up, cool down and time for stretching.

Monday	Upper Body + 30 minutes Cardio
Tuesday	Lower Body + 30 minutes Cardio
Wednesday	40 minutes Cardio + Core workout
Thursday	Full Body Strength training
Friday	Day off or yoga
Saturday	30-45 minutes Cardio
Sunday	Day Off

CREATING YOUR OWN WORKOUT ROUTINE

Use the following grid to write down your own workout plan for the week. Each week, follow the same basic format, remembering to make modifications based on your increasing fitness level. Although you can and should use the sample workouts in the previous chapter, it is a good idea to write each and every exercise you plan to perform. Keep notes on how many sets and reps you do and the weight you are using. You should be aiming for at least 2-3 strength training sessions per week and 3-5 aerobic workouts, plus stretching.

MONDAY	
TUESDAY	
WEDNESDAY	
THURSDAY	
FRIDAY	
SATURDAY	
SUNDAY	

PART THREE

Notice that Part 3 is not called *Dieting*! There are so many negative connotations and confusion over terms such as "diets" and "dieting,". It is best to consider your new outlook as a common sense approach to giving your body what it needs, just like fueling your car. Most people start diets with good intentions and a desire to stay "on track." But their motivation and any positive results they may experience typically do not last for long. The reason? Most diets set you up to fail right from the beginning because they do not provide practical, long-term solutions to weight loss or weight management. They usually have strict rules like items to eat, when to eat, and how much to eat. The vast majority of popular diets do not make allowances for personal food preferences, individual health concerns, and time constraints. They also require followers to make radical, immediate lifestyle changes that are virtually impossible to stick to for more than a few days or weeks. While they have a lot of rules, they rarely teach you the basics of eating right.

The next few chapters will teach you how to see food as an enjoyable way to prolong your life and health. Food is not something to obsess over, feel guilty about, or use as an emotional crutch. By incorporating a few simple principles into your daily routine, you can make drastic changes in both how you look and feel. But before we talk about how to develop your new eating plan, let's dispel common myths that may be keeping you from having a healthy relationship with food.

FAD DIETS

The Grapefruit Diet, the Hollywood Diet, the 3 Day Diet... these are just a few of the hundreds of fad diets that have become popular over the years. While these diets may look different, they all have one thing in common: THEY DON'T WORK! Sure, if you eat nothing but cabbage soup for a week, you may lose a few pounds, but what will happen the next week when you go back to your regular eating habits? That's right - you'll gain it all back. In fact, you may feel so deprived that you eat even more than usual and pack on some additional pounds. Here are some ways to immediately spot a fad diet:

- It relies heavily on just one food or type of food, like the above mentioned grapefruit or cabbage plans. These diets do not supply nearly enough nutrients and leave you feeling tired and miserable, not to mention totally distracted. You'll spend all of your time craving the food you miss. If you stay on these diets long enough, they could lead to dangerous nutritional deficiencies and illnesses, but that rarely happens because they are nearly impossible to stick to for more than a week.

- It bans certain foods or even entire food groups. These include high protein/low carb diets and no-fat diets. Like the single food diets, these diets do not supply all of the nutrients your body needs. Warning signs include rules that forbid foods that are good for you, like fruit and whole grains.

- It relies on prepackaged drinks, bars, or meals. An example is the Hollywood Diet, which requires followers to buy its premixed juice. A healthy diet includes a variety of fresh, unprocessed foods. Health does not come exclusively in a bottle or can. The choices on these diets are usually so limited that you will quickly become bored.

- It promises a quick fix. Phrases like "sheds pounds," "lose 10 pounds in seven days," and "melts inches" are red flags.

- Plans based on junk science. Usually these diets draw overly simplistic conclusions from complex, ongoing research or devise recommendations based on a single study.

- Diets that do not acknowledge differences among individuals or groups

HIGH PROTEIN/LOW CARB DIETS

High protein diets may be very popular right now, but they are not new. They first became popular during the 1960s and 70s, but gradually fell out of favor as the low-fat craze took over the spotlight. It is true that a lot of people do lose weight initially on high protein diets, mostly because they end up limiting the amount of food that is eaten. However, they may be harmful to your health. Not consuming adequate carbohydrates will send your body into a ketogenic state that forces it to rely on stored fat for energy. This might sound like a good thing, but it may place severe strain on your liver and kidneys.

Another problem with many high protein diets is that they encourage you to consume as many high fat foods as you want. Years of research has shown that a diet high in saturated fat can lead to heart disease, osteoporosis, some forms of cancer, diabetes, and kidney stones. Even worse, the foods banned on high protein diets, namely fruits, whole grains and some vegetables, protect your body against these ailments. Many studies have concluded that protein diets do not result in more weight loss than other calorie-restriction plans.

High protein diets work on the belief that insulin, not too many calories, makes you fat. Advocates of this type of eating maintain that when you eat too many carbs, your insulin does not effectively transport sugar to your cells and leads to more sugar being stored as fat. There is research available that both supports and debunks this theory. However, many experts firmly believe that the initial quick weight loss experienced on high protein diets is not worth the long term consequences of eating too much fat and not enough of the essential nutrients found in carbohydrates.

SO WHAT SHOULD YOU EAT?

The answer is just about anything IN MODERATION. Carbohydrates are not bad for you. Protein is not bad for you. Fat is not bad for you. Eating too much of any of them will lead to weight gain. Whether you maintain, gain, or lose weight all depends on how many calories you take in each day. When someone says they eat healthy but are still overweight, it usually comes down to portion size. You can eat healthy, but if you eat more calories than you need, you WILL gain weight.

Figuring out about how many calories you need is easy. Take your current weight in pounds and divide it by 2.2. This is your weight in kilograms. Now if you are a man, take this number and multiply it by 24 and add 200. Women should take their weight in kilograms and multiply it by 23 and then add 200. Here are some examples:

Man: 170lb / 2.2 = 77 kilograms
77 x 24 = 1848
1848 + 200 = 2048 calories per day

Woman: 140 lb / 2.2 = 64
64 x 23 = 1472
1472 + 200 = 1672 calories per day

In the above examples, the man would have to consume 2048 calories if he wanted to maintain his current weight. The woman would have to eat 1672. If these individuals wanted to lose weight, they would have to consume fewer calories.

Generally speaking, it takes 3,500 calories to create a pound of fat. Usually, it is safe and realistic to strive to lose about one to two pounds per week. You can do this by cutting about 500 calories a day from your diet or by burning an equal amount of calories through exercise. Never go under 1200 calories unless directed by a doctor. If your goal is to increase your weight, simply eat more than the number of calories you body requires for maintenance.

However, calories are only one component of maintaining a healthy lifestyle. After all, any diet, will lead to weight loss if it creates a calorie deficit. You could eat nothing but candy bars and if at the end of the day you consistently ate less calories than your body needs, you would drop pounds. But it would not take long for your health to suffer. So, if you want to lose weight, the goal is simply to reduce calories. However, if you want to be healthier (hopefully, this is your main goal), you'll need to understand how your body uses food. The next few chapters will explain how carbohydrates, protein, and fat all affect your body.

BUTT KICKIN': Calculate your caloric needs:

Weight in Pounds _____ / 2.2 = _____ x 23 (women) 24 (men) = _____

My daily caloric need to maintain my current weight is: _____

To lose 2 pounds a week I should consume: _____ calories (above minus 500)

To gain 1 pound per week I should consume: _____ calories (above +500)

CARBOHYDRATES

Carbohydrates are important because they are your body's main source of energy. They also provide the bulk of the vitamins, minerals, and fiber that you need. The trick is to pick the right carbohydrates, because they are not all created equally. Try to avoid consuming many simple carbs. Simple carbs are found in sugary foods, like candy, soft drinks, juice and processed grains, such as white flour. While these foods provide immediate energy, they also spike blood glucose levels. This is where the old cliché "what goes up, must come down" really hits you. When your blood glucose levels shoot up, you'll feel an increased level of energy, commonly known as a "sugar buzz". When your glucose levels drop, they drop fast. The crash will leave you feeling tired and hungry. Simple carbs also rarely provide fiber and nutrients. While it is fine to indulge occasionally, it is a good idea to avoid simple carbohydrates when possible.

Complex carbohydrates do not digest as quickly. Complex carbs are found in vegetables, fruits, and whole grains. Even though complex carbohydrates will eventually be converted into sugar, they do not provide a rush or a crash. Foods that are mostly made of complex carbs are also more likely to be full of fiber, vitamins and minerals, and low in fat.

The National Academy of Sciences recommends eating at least 120 grams of carbs each day (compared to popular low carb diets which allow only 20 grams a day.) Reduced carbohydrate programs like The Zone limit carbs to 40% of your diet, with the other 60% equally divided between protein and fat. However, most people find counting carbohydrates time consuming and nearly impossible, unless they have a food label in front of them. Fortunately, you don't need to count every carbohydrate to eat a healthy diet. You just have to eyeball what's on your plate. You can avoid over consuming carbohydrates with these simple principles:

First and foremost, always strive to avoid simple carbohydrates like sugar and white flour when possible. They are empty calories, meaning they provide little nutrients for the amount of fuel they provide.

Fill you plate with as many vegetables as possible and eat a liberal amount of fruit. Aim for ten ½ cup servings of fruits and vegetables a day. That may sound like a lot, but if you replace much of the junk you eat with healthy food, you'll see just how quick those servings add up.

It is fine to eat some bread and pasta in moderation. Whenever possible, substitute whole grain products for products that are made with white flour or corn meal. Whole grains, like barley, oatmeal, brown rice, and whole wheat flour provide many more nutrients and fiber. However, this does not mean you should switch to whole-wheat bread and then feel free to eat five slices with dinner. Low calorie, high volume vegetables provide many more nutrients.

BUTT KICKIN': List five complex carbohydrates you can enjoy on a daily basis.

1. _____

2. _____

3. _____

4. _____

5. _____

PROTEIN

Proteins are the building blocks of our bodies. They are comprised of 20 amino acids, which fortify our muscles, blood, skin, and internal organs. Out of these 20 acids, 12 are produced by our bodies. These are called non-essential amino acids. The other eight, called essential amino acids, have to be consumed through food and/or supplements. Both types of amino acids are necessary for our bodies to function.

Because protein builds muscle, many people try to increase their intake as a way to create more muscle while losing weight. Protein shakes, bars, and supplements are very popular and many people swear by the results. It is a fact that during resistance training and long workouts, your muscles break down and you body may benefit from an increased intake of protein. Some studies have shown that people who workout heavily may need up to 100% more protein than the current government recommendations. However, most people in the United States get more than enough protein each day and many sedentary people eat way too much protein. Basically, the more you workout, the more protein you body will need to function at optimal levels. So, how much do *you* need?

Calculate your protein needs by dividing your weight in pounds by 2.2. The resulting number is your weight in kilograms. Now, take this number and multiply it by .08 and 1.8. These two numbers are the amount of protein you body requires under different conditions. Use the first number if you are sedentary. Pregnant women, people under stress, those recovering from an illness, and those who consistently lift weights or engage in endurance training will be closer to the higher number. These populations need between 1 and 1.8. For example, 160 lb man would figure out his requirements this way:

160 / 2.2 = 72.72 kg

72.72 x 0.8 (sedentary) = 58 grams of protein

72 x 1.8 (very active) = 130 grams of protein

If he exercises regularly and lifts weights, but does not take part in endurance or power lifting activities, he will probably need somewhere around 100-110 grams of protein per day. As you can see, for the average person, this is not an exact science. Most experts recommend that your protein intake fall between 15 and 30 percent of the total number of calories you consume each day.

BUTT KICKIN': How much protein do I need on a daily basis?

1) How active are you? Sedentary = 0.8, Moderate 1.3, Active 1.8

My weight _____ divided by 2.2 = _____ Weight in kg

_____ weight in kg x ____ (activity level from above) = _____ grams of protein needed daily.

FAT AND ALCOHOL

Fat has really earned a bad reputation over the last few decades. Remember the years of the low-fat craze? Yet, while sales of low-fat products skyrocketed, the average American's waistline just kept getting bigger. That's because people who stick to a strict low-fat diet only get it half right. Some fats are bad for you, but a lot of fats are important to our bodies.

About 20% of the calories you consume each day should come from fat. Out of that fat, less than 5% should be made up of unhealthy trans and saturated fats. These fats increase your LDL, also known as "bad cholesterol" and put you at risk of heart disease. The best way to avoid these bad fats is to read the labels on the foods you eat. Saturated fat is clearly listed. The U.S. Food and Drug Administration also requires trans fatty acids appear on labels. If labels are not available, you can still avoid saturated fats by staying away from palm oil, fatty cuts of meat, butter, and high-fat dairy products, such as whole milk and cheese. Trans-fats can be harder to spot, but you'll eliminate most of them simply by cutting out processed foods. Any processed food made with partially hydrogenated vegetable oils is bound to contain trans fats. This includes cookies, candy, fried food, and even a lot of crackers.

Diets that are high in omega-3 fatty acids (the good fat) can help prevent heart disease, diabetes, and obesity, and even ease the pain of arthritis. Cold-water fish, like salmon and mackerel and canola oil (not vegetable oil) are good sources of omega 3s. Other good fat choices include nuts, olives and olive oil, tofu and soy products, and avocados.

If you are still confused about which fats are OK, put them to the solid test. Fats that are liquid at room temperature are better for you than fats that are solid at room temperature. For example, lard, shortening, and butter are all solid at room temperature, and therefore high in saturated fats. Shortening can be confusing, because it is made from what might have been healthy oil. However, it has been hydrogenated to lengthen its shelf life. The hydrogenation creates a saturated fat. Look at ingredients on labels. If you see hydrogenated or partially-hydrogenated oil, pass on it.

Alcohol falls into its own category. It supplies a lot of calories, but few nutrients. A 5-ounce glass of wine has 100 calories and 12 ounces of regular beer supplies 150 calories. Although some studies have suggested that consuming alcohol may benefit the heart, it should only be consumed in limited amounts. Generally, women should not have more than one drink per day. Men should not exceed two.

BUTT KICKIN': As the prior chapters have explained, moderation is the key to healthy eating. At each meal, try to consume mostly complex carbohydrates, especially fruits and vegetables. Then add some lean protein and some good fat.

Your Daily Calorie requirements to maintain: _____

Your Daily Calorie requirements to reduce weight: _____

Your Daily Protein Requirements: _____

Your Daily Carbohydrate Requirements: _____

SMALL CHANGES/BIG IMPROVEMENTS

By now, your head might be swimming with numbers and calculations. While these numbers may be helpful, you can also control what you eat without counting calories and grams by practicing some basic habits. Some of these tips will seem like small, easy changes. Others might take a much longer time to incorporate into your daily life. These tips will add up to large improvements in your quest to reduce your waistline and overall health.

Don't skip breakfast. Your body has already fasted during the night. It needs food to jumpstart your metabolism. Try to make breakfast a nutritionally important meal by eating some protein, a little good fat, and complex carbohydrates.

Most of the volume of food on your plate should be in the form of complex carbohydrates. However, those carbs should come mostly from fruits and vegetables. Try to limit your servings of grain based products, like bread and pasta.

> **DON'T SKIP BREAKFAST**

See each meal as a chance to do something good for yourself. Each meal, not just breakfast, should include some low-fat protein, complex carbs and a dash of healthy fats. If you aren't sure about how to do this, mentally divide your plate into half, then one side in half again. Fill one quarter with your protein. It should not be much larger than the size or thickness of your palm. Fill the other quarter with a complex carbohydrate like sweet potato or brown rice, then the remaining half of the plate with vegetables and a small amount of fat.

Become a grazer. Eat smaller meals throughout the day instead of three large meals. Never try to let more than four hours go by without eating something. It is best to eat a small meal before you are hungry, that way you will not be tempted to overeat.

Don't eat in front of the television. You may be so distracted that you just keep shoving down food without realizing that you are full. Take some time to enjoy your food and be mindful of what you are putting in your body.

As soon as you have finished eating, go brush and floss your teeth. Not only does this make for great oral hygiene, you'll be far less tempted to eat more. Toothpaste makes cookies taste terrible!

Just don't buy junk food! If you don't have it, you won't eat it. Many parents say they have to buy chips and sodas for their family, but why is this? Do growing children really need to eat garbage? Do yourself and your family a favor and purchase mostly whole, unprocessed foods. It floors me when I hear parents tell me that their kids won't eat healthy food. They will if there isn't another option. Learn to cook healthy food in a way that appeals to them. They deserve good health too. And you deserve to be in an environment that will not derail your fitness goals.

Now that you have stopped buying junk, keep cut up fruit and vegetables, low fat string cheese, and soy lunch "meat" (you may be surprised how delicious it is!) in the refrigerator. This way, all snacking is high in nutritional value and low in calories.

Learn how to read food labels. Keep a close eye on portion size and know how many servings you are eating. Stay away from foods that are high in sodium or heavily processed.

Don't fall into the "low-fat" trap. Low fat food is often high in sugar and calories to make it taste tolerable. You may be tempted to overeat if you think that eating low fat means you can eat more. Remember a calorie is still a calorie no matter how you dress it up.

Most importantly, give yourself some credit. Utilize your common sense. By now you basically know what is good for you and what foods are best avoided. Remember, you are stronger than that bowl of ice cream. Just say "no" to sabotaging your good health! More importantly recognize there will be good days and bad. Don't let one bad day derail you. Recognize where the problem is, learn from it and move on towards your goal.

BUTT KICKIN': Pantry Raid. Go through your cupboards and pantry. Look at all the labels and determine what can be removed permanently from your house so you aren't tempted.

Top Five Items Found:

1. _____

2. _____

3. _____

4. _____

5. _____

SAMPLE EATING PLAN

Now that you have some general guidelines of what to eat, I'm going to give you a little kick start to help you get off your butt and start eating healthier. Below is a sample meal plan for seven days which will get you started. Ideally you will develop a meal plan each week and stick with that plan. This will keep you from making impulse decisions on what to eat, which usually are not good choices.

Calculate your portion sizes based on the calculations you performed in previous chapters.

Day 1

Breakfast: Egg Beaters, Cream of Wheat, Cup of Blueberries, Skim Milk

AM Snack: Cottage Cheese and Cup of Sliced Peaches (fresh)

Lunch: Tuna Salad (light mayo) on Whole Wheat Pita Bread, Small Side Salad with Vinaigrette dressing on the side

PM Snack: Meal Replacement Protein Shake

Dinner: Grilled Rosemary Chicken Breast, Brown Rice, Grilled Asparagus

Day 2

Breakfast: All Bran Cereal, Unsweetened Almond Milk, Fresh Blueberries

AM Snack: Greek Strained Yogurt, ½ Whole Wheat Bagel

Lunch: Fajita Check Wrap w/ Whole Wheat Tortilla, Spanish Rice, Small Salad

PM Snack: Fruit and Chicken Bowl (Diced Chicken with Apples, Pears, Grapes and Graprefruit.)

Dinner: Broiled Tilapia w/ Lemon Pepper Seasoning, green beans and smashed red potatoes (use chicken broth)

Day 3

Breakfast: 2 Hard Boiled Eggs (1 Yolk), Oatmeal, ½ Banana

AM Snack: Whole Wheat Crakers, 2% Colby Cheese (reduced fat)

Lunch: Chicken Salad with Whole Wheat Bagel, Small Salad

PM Snack: Non-Fat, No Sugar Added Yogurt and Fresh Peach

Dinner: Chicken Stir Fry w/ Fresh Vegetables and Low Sodium Soy Sauce over Brown Rice

Day 4

Breakfast: All Bran Cereal, 2 Hard Boiled Eggs, Unsweetened Almond Milk, ½ Grapefruit

AM Snack: Yogurt w/ Granola

Lunch: Turkey Breast Sandwich on Whole Wheat Bagel w/ Sliced Tomato and Spinach, Sweet Potato Baked Fries

PM Snack: Almonds and Apple

Dinner: Broiled Salmon, Spinach Salad, Mashed Sweet Potatoes

Day 5

Breakfast: 3 Scrambled Egg Whites, Oatmeal, Fresh Strawberries

AM Snack: Bagel and Fat Free Cream Cheese

Lunch: Baked Potato with Ground Turkey Meat and Salsa, Small Side Salad

PM Snack:	Raw Strawberries, 8 oz Almond Milk – Unsweetened
Dinner:	No Sugar Added BBQ Sauce on Pork Tenderloin, Green Beans, roasted Red Potatoes

Day 6

Breakfast:	All Bran Cereal, Unsweetened Almond Milk, Fresh Blueberries
AM Snack:	Yogurt w/ Granola
Lunch:	Chicken Salad with Whole Wheat Bagel, Small Salad
PM Snack:	Meal Replacement Protein Shake
Dinner:	Broiled Flank Steak (lean), Corn Tortillas, Salsa, Avocado Slice, Small Salad

Day 7

Breakfast:	2 Hard Boiled Eggs (1 Yolk), Oatmeal, ½ Banana
AM Snack:	Whole Wheat Crakers, 2% Colby Cheese (reduced fat)
Lunch:	Tuna Salad (light mayo) on Whole Wheat Pita Bread, Small Side Salad with Vinaigrette dressing on the side
PM Snack:	Raw Strawberries, 20 Raw Almonds
Dinner:	Broiled Tilapia w/ Lemon Pepper Seasoning, green beans and baked sweet potato cubes.

BUTT KICKIN': With this sample menu plan you can now start to create your own menu plans using your own recipes. The key to being successful is planning. Without a plan you are more likely to make bad choices with your food.

Log on the **www.GetOffYourButtNDoSomething.com** and download the meal planning template in the resources section.

My First Week Menu Plan

Day 1:

Day 2:

Day 3:

Day 4:

Day 5

Day 6:

Day 7:

EMOTIONAL EATING

Did you just read the *Small Changes/Big Improvements* section of the book and think, "Yeah, but (fill in blank)..." For many of us, eating is about far more than giving our body the energy it needs to sustain itself. Starting in our childhoods, we are rewarded with food. Think of all of those ice cream cones after a baseball game or cookies given to soothe scraped knees. In a culture where food is so often seen as love, it makes sense that we have a hard time putting its role in our life into proper perspective. Getting over emotional eating is a major battle for most people struggling to control their weight.

The emotions that prompt people into overeating are complicated and deep-seeded. You may reach for chocolate when you feel sad. You may mindlessly snack on chips when you are feeling bored or stressed out. Perhaps you feel the need to clean your plate as a way to show appreciation toward the loved one who cooked the meal. Whatever your reasons, you will have to become more aware of what you are eating and why you do it if you want to conquer emotional eating. Keep a journal or make a list of the situations when you eat to fill an emotional need. Identify the times you are most likely to get off track.

Now start to realize something that is very important: Other people may affect your emotions, but only you are responsible for what you put in your mouth. You must be accountable for what you eat. You will not always be able to keep emotional eating in check, but unless you acknowledge your complex feelings about food, you cannot make any real changes. Understanding what leads you to overeating will make it easier to form new coping strategies and healthy eating habits.

BUTT KICKIN': What Are Your Emotional Triggers?

1. _____

2. _____

3. _____

WATER

Our bodies are more than 60% water. Muscles, lungs, and brains contain a lot of water and our blood is almost entirely water. The water in our body regulates our temperature and is the medium that carries nutrients throughout our body, while carrying waste away from our tissues. It is important to consume enough water because we constantly lose fluid throughout the day. Water is lost primarily through sweating, urinating, and even breathing. Now that you have started your path to fitness you'll have to be mindful of how much fluid you consume. You lose so much more water when exercising. This is especially true if you take-in diuretics, like caffeine or certain medications, that may lead to increased water loss.

> OUR BODIES ARE MORE THAN 60% WATER

Although thirst is an obvious sign of dehydration, it is not advisable to drink only when you are thirsty. Unfortunately, thirst comes after the fact, so by the time you feel thirsty, you are already dehydrating. Other symptoms of dehydration include headaches, constipation, lower back pain, and achy joints and muscles. You can easily tell if you are dehydrated by looking at your urine. A strong odor or yellow color is an indication that your body needs water.

Just how much water you should drink everyday has been the subject of great debate. For years, people were told to drink eight glasses a day, but that thinking has changed somewhat. Experts now recognize that the need for water varies among individuals, depending on size and activity level. A simple way to determine how much water you need is to take your weight and divide it in half. That is the number of ounces of water each day you should try to drink. Eight ounces equals one cup, so a 150 pound person would need 75 ounces of fluid, or about 9 cups of water a day. On days you exercise, try to drink about another cup of water for each 20 minutes of activity. People who live in especially dry climates may need a few additional servings a day.

The best way to get water is to simply drink it plain. Get in the habit of filling up a big bottle of water to keep nearby while you are working. Take the bottle with you when you are traveling or working out. If you find the taste of water unpalatable, adding lemon juice can make it more flavorful. Try to avoid meeting your fluid needs with soft drinks or juices because they are full of sugar. If you enjoy the taste of sports drinks, they may be a good choice, but look at the label to make sure they are not full of empty calories or excess carbohydrates.

BUTT KICKIN': How much water should I have on a daily basis?

My weight in pounds _____

Divided by 2 = _____ oz of water I should consume daily.

SLEEP

Sleep is a crucial part of maintaining a healthy lifestyle. No matter how well you eat or exercise, you will never feel or function at your best as long as you are chronically tired. Yet, despite all of the warnings about not getting enough sleep, we still tend to shortchange ourselves each night. For adults, anything less than seven hours of sleep a night is asking for trouble. Some people, including pregnant women and the elderly, may require even more rest. Contrary to popular belief, you cannot train yourself to need less sleep. Your body never gets used to being tired. No matter how you rationalize it, do not try to convince yourself that you are somehow able to get by on only four hours a night. Unless you have some kind of rare genetic makeup, you are kidding yourself.

Lack of sleep often leads to a list of problems. Proper rest is necessary for our nervous systems to function. Memory, concentration, coordination, mood and energy levels are all directly tied to your level of sleep. Lack of sleep may also lead to weight gain! Scientists are still trying to figure out why people with sleep problems (especially sleep apnea) are more prone to obesity. It may be due to the hormones that regulate food intake. There is also evidence that not getting enough deep sleep can reduce the levels of an important growth hormone that regulates how much fat and muscle your body creates.

Studies have shown that women are more likely than men to suffer sleep deprivation. The reasons are complex and may include everything from household and career demands to hormone fluctuations associated with pregnancy and menopause. In fact, some research has shown that nearly two-thirds of American women are getting less than eight hours of sleep a night!

It is imperative that you make sleep a top priority if you are truly committed to improving your quality of life. However, it is normal to go through periods when you will not get adequate sleep. Hopefully, if you are experiencing insomnia, it will only last a few days at a time. If chronic sleeping problems affect you, seek treatment. Your doctor may help you pinpoint the cause and develop an effective course of treatment. Treatment may include reconditioning and relaxation therapy. Remember, sleep is not a luxury or an indulgence. It is essential to keeping you strong and happy.

WEIGHT LOSS SUPPLEMENTS

You are probably reading this book because you want to permanently lose weight, gain strength, and be the healthiest you can be. If that is the case, don't ever resort to weight loss supplements. Let me repeat that in case you didn't read it right the first time.. **DON'T EVER RESORT TO WEIGHT LOSS PILLS**!! It's not worth it! Weight loss pills have been proven time and time again to be dangerous. Period... end of story.

Of course, the ads are tempting. Who doesn't want to see pounds "disappear?" Plus, the marketing ploys often show people who claim to be satisfied customers. They are smiling and armed with impressive before and after photographs. Some weight loss pill companies even offer a money back guarantees. Don't fall for these tricks.

Yes, it is true that some pills may help you lose a little weight, but when you stop taking the pills the weight comes right back. So, what's the point? Even scarier is the fact that many of the supplements available are not well regulated and may have questionable ingredients. In some cases, the pills might be dangerous. For instance, the government banned ephedra in 2003 because of serious concerns about its safety. Ephedra is gone, but there are similar compounds on the market. They present the same dangers as ephedra, including seizures, stroke, and heart attacks. Unless you are 100% sure you know what you are taking and you have cleared it with your doctor, it is not a good idea to take weight loss supplements. Common sense eating and exercise are the only sure-fire, risk-free way to shed pounds and improve your health.

YO-YO DIETING AND YOUR METABOLISM

Yo-yo dieting is a common term for a very common problem. It happens when people lose a lot of weight through dieting and then gain it all back, only to lose it again. You may have heard people say that years of yo-yo dieting have forever ruined their metabolism (the rate at which your bodies burn calories.) This is a myth. Although yo-yo dieting does adversely affect your metabolism, you can overcome the problem and get your body back on track.

> CELLULITE IS JUST FAT! YOU CAN'T SPOT REDUCE IT!

When you lose a lot of weight through crash diets, much of what you are losing is muscle. If you pack the pounds back on fairly quickly once the diet is over, the new weight will almost always be in the form of fat. You may end up weighing the same as you did before you went on the diet, but your body composition is now very different. The percentage of your body that is fat may have skyrocketed. This is where yo-yo dieting creates problems with your metabolic rate.

As we have already discussed, your muscles are responsible for most of the calories your body uses for energy. Take away a lot of muscle and you've lost some of your capacity to burn those calories. You'll gain even more fat if you have returned to your old eating habits. The effect of yo-yo dieting on your metabolism can be reversed by building muscle through strength training. As you regain the muscle you have lost, your body will burn more calories, even during periods of rest. Once you start exercising and stop "dieting" by making healthy eating an ingrained part of your lifestyle, you'll be able to boost your metabolism and put yo-yo dieting behind you forever.

CELLULITE

It's been called orange peel skin, hail damage and cottage cheese thighs. No matter what you call it, women are in a never ending battle to get rid of cellulite. Cellulite is lumps and bumps that show up in varying degrees on the thighs and hips of nearly 85% of women.

Companies have made a lot of money selling women creams, wraps, and pills that promise to flush out that pesky fat. Unfortunately, desperate women who try the so-called cures just end up with less money and the same old fat. Getting rid of cellulite is the same as trying to "spot reduce." Your body just doesn't work that way. So stop obsessing with the cellulite and start obsessing about eating right and exercising routinely.

There is nothing special about cellulite. It is just plain fat. It forms when pockets of fat are attached to fibrous tissue. The skin is pulled in, the fat is pushed out, and the result is those dimples that make women cringe. How much cellulite you have is largely influenced by genetics, hormonal changes, and of course, gaining weight.

If you battle with cellulite, you already know how tough it is to destroy. Some women will always have cellulite, no matter how hard they try to fight it. However, there are steps you can take to minimize its appearance. Stop smoking and limit caffeine. There is some evidence that both may make cellulite look worse since they constrict blood vessels. The biggest improvements will come through healthy eating and consistent exercise. This winning combination will reduce the amount of fat you have throughout your entire body, including on your hips and thighs.

PART FOUR

Congratulations! You now have the tools to build a stronger, healthier body. Once you start seeing positive changes, you'll understand the power of exercise and nutrition and feel even more motivated to keep going. However, there will be times that working out or eating well just will not happen. Don't beat yourself up about it. Simply move on to the next day and try to do better. Reaching your personal fitness goals is often a long journey, full of twists and turns. But if you stay on track as much as possible, you'll achieve your goals. When I first started my quest for fitness I was clueless and would try something for 2 weeks and quit. What I've outlined in this book works, it has for the hundreds of clients I've personally coached and it can work for you to. We all basically know what we need to do, it's the implementation which is the difficult part.

When you have been working out for a few weeks, you might start to feel like your routine is becoming monotonous. If that is the case, immediately change it! Not only will change keep your workouts from getting boring, it will increase your level of fitness. Your muscles quickly adapt to the stress you put on them and they stop growing. It's good to shock them every few weeks with a new routine. A new program can be as simple as increasing the amount of weight you are using by a safe amount or performing more repetitions. You may also want to try different exercises and machines for each body part.

Just as you may get bored with a workout routine, eventually you may need to incorporate new foods into your diet. Often people cut out a long list of unhealthy foods and replace them with only a few healthy choices. Eating the same meals and snacks over and over will get tiresome and may make you more prone to cheating. Variety in your diet is also crucial to getting enough nutrients. Try to incorporate new foods into your meal plans every week. Trying out a new type of fish or exotic fruits and vegetables will help keep things interesting. You may even discover new favorites.

Don't forget about your initial fitness assessment. Keep your measurements, weight, and endurance and strength test results with your exercise calendar. Chart your progress at least every four weeks. Nothing feels as good as seeing real progress. Of course, you may not always see the results you want. That's OK. Use the information to analyze and modify your routine. You should be able to get the numbers moving in the right direction again. Once you have reached your goals, still take the time for a full assessment at least every three months to make sure you are holding steady.

Good luck as you embark on your wonderful new lifestyle. You deserve to be as healthy and fit as possible. It is the best gift you will ever give yourself. Sometimes the progress will be fast. Other times it will seem way too slow. Just remember there are no magic foods, pills, or supplements that can do as much for your body as eating a balanced, healthy diet and maintaining a consistent program of aerobic, strength and flexibility training.

Check out the many resources available at this book's website: www.GetOffYourButtNDoSomething.com

Don't Wait Until It's Too Late To Get Off Your Butt and Do Something and Regain Your Attractive, Healthy, Energetic Body Once And For All!

Tom's Kick-Start Trial Enrollment Form
Just $297
save over $200
Limited Time Offer
(only valid for new clients)

❑ *YES!* I'm excited to work with Body3 Fitness Center, and have you demonstrate how personal training can benefit me. I know you'll be there to hold my hand through all the obstacles I've encountered in the past (but could never breakthrough), and show me the quickest, easiest and most effective route to getting the strong, lean, healthy body I've always wanted!

I can't wait to pick your brain and learn your "insider" health and fitness secrets during each of the 8 30-minute private training sessions which I will schedule as well as the initial health and fitness evaluation and consultation.

I understand you'll teach me all the **proven systems and strategies** you've developed over the years to get dramatic, life-changing results with all your private clients. And because I'm serious about getting those kind of results for myself, I'm not going to wait a moment longer to reserve one of the 10 LIMITED SPOTS available for this special offer which will include...

- **8 personal training sessions over 1 month** where I'll work with a fitness trainer one-on-one to make sure I stay on the fastest track to getting the results I want and desire.
- **1 Nutrition and health consultation** at which I will learn tips and tricks to optimize the way I eat so I'm fueling my body correctly and appropriately for my new activity level.
- **1-Month Full Access to Body3 Fitness Center** where I can take high energy group fitness classes like, BodyCombat, BodyPump, BodyFlow, or Zumba.

I'm ready to share my newfound health and fitness with my family and friend! I can't wait to feel healthy, confident and happy about my body... and I know if I follow your **proven system**, I will be successful!

❑ No thanks, the kick-start program isn't for me. But I am interested in more information about your programs, including **Pilates, group training, boot camp, or membership**. Please contact me to schedule a complimentary private consultation with you *($75 value)*.

Name: _____ Date: _____ Birth Date: _____

Address: _____

City: _____ State: _____ Zip Code: _____

Email: _____

Home #: _____ Mobile: _____

Email to: support @Body3Fit.com

www.ingramcontent.com/pod-product-compliance
Lightning Source LLC
Chambersburg PA
CBHW020312290526
45784CB00003B/1486